Pocket Guide to
Respiratory Care

Pocket Guide to Respiratory Care

Pamela Becker Weilitz, RN, MSN (R)
Pulmonary Clinical Nurse Specialist
Barnes Hospital
St. Louis, Missouri

Illustrated

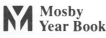

Mosby
Year Book

St. Louis   Baltimore   Boston   Chicago   London   Philadelphia   Sydney   Toronto

M Mosby
Year Book

Editor: Don Ladig
Developmental Editor: Robin Carter
Assistant Editor: Kathleen Higley
Project Supervisor: Barbara Merritt
Design: Laura Steube

COVER ART © Ron Boisvert

Printed in the United States of America

Mosby–Year Book, Inc
11830 Westline Industrial Drive, St. Louis, Missouri 63146

Library of Congress Cataloging-in-Publication Data

Weilitz, Pamela Becker

Pocket guide to respiratory care / Pamela Becker Weilitz.

p.   cm.
Includes bibliographical references.
Includes index.
ISBN 0-8016-0189-4
1. Respiratory organs—Diseases—Nursing—Handbooks, manuals, etc.
I. Title.
[DNLM: 1. Respiration Disorders—nursing—handbooks. WY 39 W422p]
RC735.5.W45   1991
610.73'692—dc20
DNLM/DLC
for Library of Congress

90-13256
CIP

C/RRD/RRD   9 8 7 6 5 4 3 2 1

To

Alan for his love and support

and to

the memory of **Jeff**

Consultant Board

Preface

Pocket Guide to Respiratory Care is designed to be a resource for nurses who provide care for clients with respiratory alterations. The text is developed using the nursing process; assessment, nursing diagnosis, planning, intervention, and evaluation, with regard to clients with acute care, home care and extended care needs.

The first chapter assesses clients with respiratory alterations. Included is a guide for completing a history and complete physical assessment of the respiratory system. Information given includes rationale for the test, significant findings, and nursing considerations.

Chapter 2 relates the formation of the nursing diagnosis. The diagnosis, related factors, and defining characteristics are presented to allow the nurse to select the appropriate nursing diagnosis based on the assessment data. Respiratory diagnoses as well as related diagnoses are presented.

Chapter 3 provides a quick reference to frequently encountered respiratory diseases. The chapter includes a descriptive summary of acute and chronic assessment findings. Nursing interventions commonly instituted are listed to assist the nurse in planning care.

Chapters 4 through 7 offer interventions for care of the respiratory client: airway management, respiratory medications, oxygenation management, and mechanical ventilation. Each chapter contains indications for the intervention, nursing responsibilities, and any special nursing considerations that may be necessary.

Chapters 8 and 9 complete the health care spectrum with details of pulmonary rehabilitation and respiratory home care. Nursing care plans, nursing interventions, and evaluation of expected outcomes assist the nurse in developing care plans for pulmonary rehabilitation and determining home care needs.

Throughout the text I have tried to provide the nurse with accurate, current, and practical information about caring for the client with respiratory alterations. I would like to acknowledge the encouragement, nurturing, and care of Dr. Myron Jacobs, Dr. Royal Eaton, and Dr. Mark Wald. Throughout the past 16 years they have shared with me their vast knowledge and love of pulmonary medicine and helped to develop my skill and love for the care of the respiratory client. I would also like to acknowledge Anne Griffin Perry, my mentor throughout graduate school and in my current practice as a clinical specialist.

Pamela Becker Weilitz

Contents

Respiratory
Assessment

1

The first step of the nursing process is *assessment*. Assessment includes the history, physical examination, and review of diagnostic data.

One of the most important parts of the assessment is obtaining an accurate and complete history. Many clients do not readily volunteer information regarding their health status. The nurse must be skilled in asking direct questions and be responsive to answers to allow additional questioning. Since many clients with respiratory problems are short of breath, direct, short-answer questions are best. Areas to interview specific to the respiratory system include breathlessness, characteristics of cough and sputum, previous respiratory illnesses, smoking history, activity level, sleep patterns, hospitalizations, oxygen therapy, intubations, and mechanical ventilation. A complete history should be taken on all clients including a review of systems, past medical-surgical history, medications, and social and familial history.

Table 1-1 identifies areas of respiratory history and suggested interview questions.

Table 1-1 Pulmonary history

Interview topics	Interview questions
Activity level	How would you describe your activity level? Active? Sedentary?
	Are you able to do the activities you would like? Shopping? Walking? Housework?
	How far can you walk? Why do you stop?
	Has your activity changed recently?
	Can you climb stairs?
Breathlessness	Are you aware of your breathing?
	Has your breathing changed? When?
	How often do you have shortness of breath?
	Does a change in position relieve or increase the shortness of breath?
	Does your breathlessness interfere with things you want to do?
Cough	Do you cough frequently?
	Does anything seem to trigger the coughing?
	How would you describe your cough?
	Do you produce much sputum? How much? How often? What color? What consistency?
	What makes your cough better?
Smoking	Have you ever smoked?
	What do/did you smoke?
	How old were you when you started? Stopped?
	How many packs per day and how many years smoked?
Respiratory illness	Have you ever been told you have lung disease? What? When?

Does your family have a history of tuberculosis, malignancy, emphysema, asthma, or chronic bronchitis?

Have you ever had pneumonia? When?

Have you ever taken steroids for your respiratory illness?

What medications do you take?

Sleep patterns

How many hours do you sleep at night?

Do you awaken frequently at night?

Do you sleep during the day? Do you snore?

How many pillows do you use at night?

Do you wake up short of breath?

Oxygen therapy

Do you use oxygen at home?

When? How much?

How long have you been using oxygen?

What type of system do you use?

Hospitalizations

When was your most recent hospitalization for respiratory illness?

How many times were you admitted in the past year?

Did you undergo intubation or mechanical ventilation? If so, what was the date and length of time?

Environmental factors

Have you ever been exposed to hazardous chemicals?

What is the nature of your work?

Are there environmental hazards? Possible allergens? Heating/air conditioning?

Do you live in an urban or rural area?

Physical Examination

Physical examination of the chest and thorax should be conducted and documented using standard chest landmarks (Fig. 1-1), enabling the nurse to localize findings and communicate them to other health care team members.

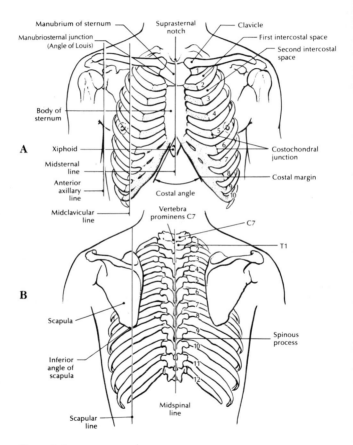

Figure 1-1

Topographic landmarks: A, Anterior thorax. B, Posterior thorax.

(From Malasanos L: Health assessment, ed 4, St Louis, 1990, The CV Mosby Co.)

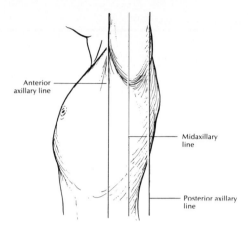

C

Figure 1-1 cont'd.
Topographic landmarks: **C**, Lateral thorax.

Inspection

Inspection begins with the overall pattern of the client's breathing. Observe the body positioning, use of accessory muscles of respiration, chest wall configuration, and respiratory pattern. Notice the shape of the chest wall. In an adult the anteroposterior diameter should be 1:2 or 5:7. Other configurations are barrel chest, pectus excavatum (funnel chest), pectus carinatum (pigeon chest), and kyphoscoliosis.

The respiratory pattern should be observed for rate, depth, and inspiratory and expiratory cycles (Table 1-2). Note whether the client is using pursed lip breathing since it improves gas exchange, increasing the PaO_2 by providing positive end expiration to the alveoli.

Observation of chest wall movement determines depth of respiration as well as symmetry of chest wall expansion. The chest wall should increase in lateral width and anteroposterior diameter during inspiration. Unequal movement suggests reduced ventilation to the affected side.

Table 1-2   Respiratory pattern

Type/Pattern	Rate (breaths per minute)	Clinical Significance
Eupnea	16-20	Normal
Tachypnea	>35	Respiratory failure Response to fever Anxiety Shortness of breath Respiratory infection
Bradypnea	<10	Sleep Respiratory depression Drug overdose Central nervous system (CNS) lesion
Apnea	Periods of no respiration lasting >15 seconds	May be intermittent such as in sleep apnea Respiratory arrest
Hypernea	16-20	Can result from anxiety or response to pain Can cause marked respiratory alkalosis, parasthesia, tetany, confusion
Kussmaul's	Usually >35, may be slow or normal	Tachypnea pattern associated with diabetic ketoacidosis, metabolic acidosis, or renal failure

Table 1-2   Respiratory pattern—cont'd

Type/Pattern	Rate (breaths per minute)	Clinical Significance
Cheyne-Stokes	Variable	Crescendo-decrescendo pattern caused by alterations in acid base status. Underlying metabolic problem or neuro-cerebral insult
Biot's	Variable	Periods of apnea and shallow breathing caused by CNS disorder; found in some healthy clients
Apneustic	Increased	Increased inspiratory time with short grunting expiratory time; seen in CNS lesions of the respiratory center

Normal muscles of respiration are the diaphragm and intercostals. Clients with respiratory alterations use the less efficient sternocleidomastoid, trapezeus, pectoral, and scalene muscles to breathe. The accessory muscles of respiration improve diaphragmatic efficiency.

Extremities are observed for color, temperature, and clubbing of the fingers (Table 1-3). Color is the most unreliable indicator of adequate oxygenation; however, it does suggest adequacy of circulation. Clients consuming nicotine will have decreased peripheral vascular circulation resulting in variable color changes and decreased temperature. Clubbing of the fingers is found in clients with chronic lung disease such as fibrosis, congenital heart disease, chronic hypoxia, or chronic obstructive lung disease (Fig. 1-2).

Table 1-3 Extremity assessment

	Alteration	Clinical Significance
Skin	Color	Peripheral vascular disease (PVD), cold, nicotine use, hypoxia
	Temperature	Fever
	Diaphoresis	Hypoxia
		Fever
		Hypotension
Fingers	Clubbing	Chronic pulmonary problem
	Nailbed cyanosis	Decreased peripheral circulation
		Hypoxia

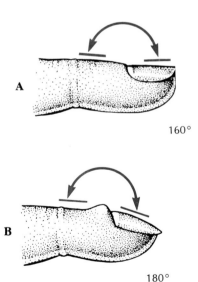

Figure 1-2
A, Normal angle of the nail. **B,** Abnormal angle of the nail seen in late clubbing.
(From Malasanos L: Health assessment, ed 4, St Louis, 1990, The CV Mosby Co.)

Palpation

Palpation is used to assess abnormalities suggested by the history or noted during inspection, such as skin and subcutaneous structures, thoracic expansion, tactile fremitus, and tracheal position. Skin is palpated for temperature and turgor. The thoracic skeleton and muscle mass are palpated for symmetry, as follows:

Thoracic Expansion

(Fig. 1-3)   Assess for equal expansion. Decrease may result from pneumonia, atelectasis, pneumothorax, pneumonectomy

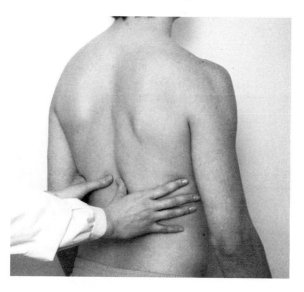

Figure 1-3
Palpation of thoracic expansion.
(From Malasanos L: Health assessment, ed 4, St Louis, 1990, The CV Mosby Co.)

Tactile Fremitus

Vibrations felt through the chest wall as the client inspires and expires. Use the palmar base of the fingers or the ulnar aspect of the hand or fist (Fig. 1-4)

Indicates increased secretions, possibly increased atelectasis or consolidation

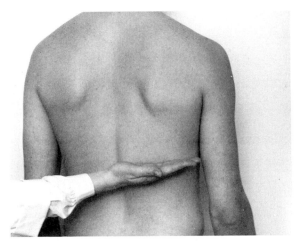

Figure 1-4
Palpation for assessment of vocal fremitus; use of ulnar aspect of the hand.
(From Malasanos L: Health assessment, ed 4, St Louis, 1990, The CV Mosby Co.)

Vocal Fremitus

Palpable vibration of thorax produced by phonation; technique same as tactile fremitus

Increased in pneumonia, lung tumor, pulmonary fibrosis.
Decreased in pleural effusion, pleural thickening, pneumothorax, bronchial obstruction, emphysema

Pleural Friction Rub

Vibration produced by inflamed pleural surfaces; felt on inspiration

Pleuritis, postpneumothorax

Crepitations

Subcutaneous emphysema (leakage of air into subcutaneous tissue) (Fig. 1-5)

Presence indicates air in the subcutaneous tissue, improperly placed tracheostomy tube, chest trauma, pleural tear, thoracic tear following invasive procedure

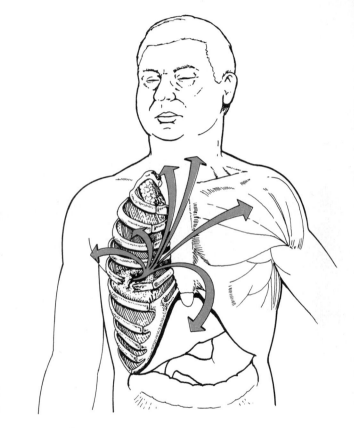

Figure 1-5
Subcutaneous emphysema.

Percussion

Percussion is the tapping of an object to determine relative amounts of air, liquid, or solid in the underlying tissue (Malasanos, 1986). Percussion is done by striking the middle finger of the nondominant hand with the middle finger of the dominant hand or a percussion hammer (Fig. 1-6). Specific sounds are heard over various parts of the body. These sounds are produced by organs that are fluid filled, air filled, and solid. Table 1-4 describes each note of percussion, where it is located, and its significance.

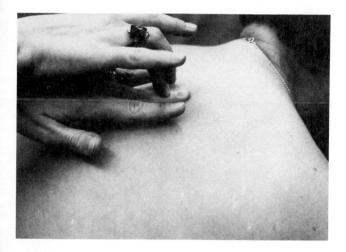

Figure 1-6
Indirect percussion. Positioning of hands.
(From Malasanos L: Health assessment, ed 4, St Louis, 1990, The CV Mosby Co.)

Table 1-4 Percussion sounds

Percussion Note	Definition	Significance
Flat	Very dense, airless tissue; soft, high pitched, brief	Normal: liver, shoulders
Dullness	Little air is present; moderately high pitched; short, soft, muffled; no musical sound	Normal: diaphragm, vertebral column, scapulae, spleen, heart
Resonance	Air-filled lungs; low pitched	Normal: lung
Hyperresonance	Resonance, louder, somewhat musical; decreased pitch	Hyperinflation, air trapping
Tympany	Completely air-filled organ	Normal: stomach when air collects between pleural space in open or closed pneumothorax
Flat or dull over lung	Conditions replacing air in alveoli with fluid or tissue	Pneumonia, pulmonary edema, atelectasis, effusions, infections

Diaphragmatic excursion

Diaphragmatic excursion is usually 3 to 5 cm. The steps to assess diaphragmatic excursion are as follows:

1. Ask client to take a deep breath.
2. Percuss the posterior thorax from superior chest wall to inferior chest wall, noting the change of sound from resonant to dull.
3. Mark point of change.
4. Ask client to exhale and resume a few normal breaths.
5. Ask client to take breath and exhale completely.
6. Percuss the thorax from inferior chest wall to superior chest wall starting at the mark on the posterior chest wall.
7. Note point of change from dull to resonant.
8. Measure excursion.
9. Instruct client to breathe normally.

The diaphragm should move equally. Unequal excursion can be the result of diaphragmatic paralysis, decreased lung expansion, or denervation of the hemi-diaphragm (Fig. 1-7).

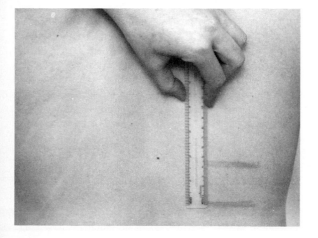

Figure 1-7

Assessment of diaphragmatic excursion.

(From Malasanos L: Health assessment, ed 4, St Louis, 1990, The CV Mosby Co.)

Auscultation (Table 1-5)

Auscultation provides information about the movement of air through the bronchial tree (Figs. 1-8 to 1-10). Auscultation is completed using the diaphragm of the stethoscope.

Oxygen Assessment (Table 1-6)

Assessment of oxygenation indicates how well oxygen is transported to the cells and includes cardiac output (CO), hemoglobin (Hgb), and the partial pressure of arterial oxygen saturation (Pao_2). The cardiac output determines how efficiently oxygen is transported to the cells. Normal CO is 4 to 6 l/min. As the carrier of the oxygen molecule, hemoglobin is capable of carrying 1.34 ml of O_2/g of hemoglobin. Arterial oxygen saturation reflects how much oxygen the hemoglobin is carrying. Oxyhemoglobin represents 98% of the overall oxygen content.

The Pao_2, which is the most frequently assessed oxygenation parameter, only reflects 2% of the total oxygen content.

Ventilation Assessment

Arterial blood gas sampling provides information about oxygenation and ventilation. Arterial blood gas reports include arterial blood pH, partial pressure of arterial oxygen, and arterial carbon dioxide, and arterial oxygen saturation. Arterial blood gas sampling begins by assessing the client's available sites. The radial and brachial arteries are preferable because of collateral circulation; relative proximity to the surface anatomy; and decreased pain from large muscle, fat, and tendon supply. The radial artery is preferable, since collateral circulation can be tested using Allen's test, as follows:

1. Have client make tight fist.
2. Apply direct pressure to both radial and ulnar arteries.
3. Have client open hand, which will be blanched.
4. Release pressure over ulnar artery; observe for return of circulation, which indicates adequate collateral flow (Fig. 1-11).

Table 1-5 Auscultation

Sound/Description	Clinical Significance	Nursing Implications
Bronchial or tracheal—hollow, blowing sound heard over large airways such as the trachea and right and left main stem bronchus	Normal; pathological if heard over smaller airways indicating airway obstruction and dilatation proximal to the obstruction; indicates pulmonary consolidation	None
Vesicular—airy, whispery sound heard over the periphery of the lung	Normal	None
Bronchovesicular—combination of vesicular and bronchial sounds heard over the smaller bronchioles; long, loud expiratory sound	Normal; if heard peripherally may indicate some consolidation	None
Adventitious Sounds		
Wheeze—continuous (>250 ms) high-pitched sound caused when the airway narrows to the point of opposite walls touching	Caused by bronchospasm, the presence of mucus, or edema of the airway diameter; can be associated with airway plugging, tumor, or foreign body	Report assessment findings; assess for shortness of breath; administer bronchodilators.

Continued.

Table 1-5   Auscultation—cont'd

Sound/Description	Clinical Significance	Nursing Implications
Crackle—discontinuous sound (20 ms); series of brief, explosive sounds; dry quality; may be heard more on inspiration	Presence of mucus, pus, or fluid in airway. **Note:** Crackles caused by cardiac failure are gravity dependent and will move throughout the thorax relative to patient positioning	Report assessment findings; determine if the crackles are pulmonary or cardiac
Rhonchus—continuous rumbling sound; may be heard more on expiration	In presence of thick secretions, external pressure, airway obstruction, or muscular spasm; frequently clears with coughing; may be associated with findings of tactile fremitus	Report assessment findings; provide chest physiotherapy/postural drainage (CPT/PD); provide pulmonary hygiene measures of suctioning, coughing, and deep breathing
Pleural friction rub—cracking, grating sound	Indicates area of pleural inflammation or roughened pleural surfaces	Report findings to physician

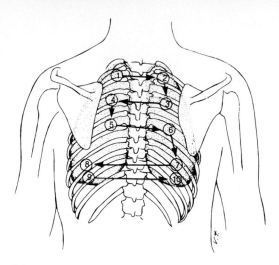

Figure 1-8
Posterior auscultation sequence.
(Perry A and Potter P: Clinical nursing skills and techniques, ed 2, St Louis, 1990, The CV Mosby Co.)

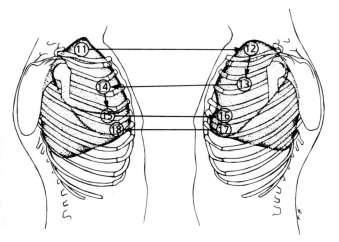

Figure 1-9
Lateral auscultation sequence.
(Perry A and Potter P: Clinical nursing skills and techniques, ed 2, St Louis, 1990, The CV Mosby Co.)

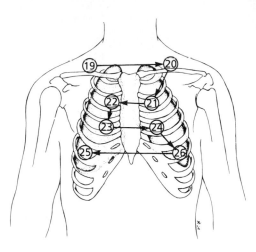

Figure 1-10
Anterior auscultation sequence.
(Perry A and Potter P: Clinical nursing skills and techniques, ed 2, St Louis, 1990, The CV Mosby Co.)

The sampling syringe should be prepared with 0.5 ml sodium heparin. The entire barrel should be washed and all but 0.15 to 0.25 ml of heparin left in the syringe should be discarded. A 23- or 25-gauge needle should be used.

The arterial sample technique is as follows:

1. Palpate and stabilize artery with gloved hands (Figs. 1-12 and 1-13).
2. Clean area with alcohol preparation.
3. Hold needle bevel up and insert at 45-degree angle.
4. Stop advancing needle when blood return is noted.
5. Withdraw 2 to 3 ml of arterial blood.
6. Remove needle and apply direct pressure to artery for 5 to 10 minutes.
7. Cap sample, expelling any air bubbles.
8. Place syringe in cup of crushed ice and transport to laboratory.

Arterial blood gases can be drawn at 10 to 15 minutes after a change in oxygen therapy. The current Fio_2 should always be included on the laboratory requisition, since this knowledge will al-

Table 1-6 Oxygenation assessment

Assessment Parameter	Formula	Significance
O_2 content (Cao_2)	$(Hgb \times 1.34 \times Sao_2) + (Pao_2 \times .003)$*	Normal 20 vols %; decrease reflects fall in oxygen supply
Oxygen transport	$Cao_2 \times CO \times 10$	600 to 100 cc/minute; decrease indicates drop in delivery of oxygen to the tissues
Alveolar air equation	$Pao_2 = Fio_2 (P_B - P_{H_2O}) - Paco_2.8$	Normal 100 mm Hg on room air
Alveolar-arterial gradient (P[A-a]o$_2$)	$PAo_2 - Pao_2$	Normal 10 mm Hg on room air; 100 mm Hg on Fio_2 100%; used to determine intrapulmonary shunt and ventilation/perfusion mismatch
Arterial/alveolar ratio (a-A ratio)	$\dfrac{Pao_2}{P_Ao_2}$	Estimates the degree of intrapulmonary shunt. Varies with $Paco_2$ and ventilation/perfusion ratios; Normal .80 Moderate shunt .50-.80 Significant shunt .25-.50 Critical shunt <.25

*Because the amount of the Pao_2 is small, many clinicians calculate the first part of the formula only.

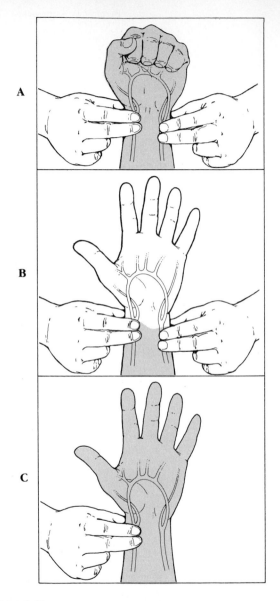

Figure 1-11
Allen test. **A,** Occlude both arteries with firm pressure. **B,** Raise arm to blanch hand. **C,** Release ulnar artery for return of color to hand.

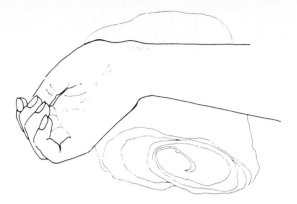

Figure 1-12
Correct position to obtain wrist extension for puncture of the radial artery. Broken line approximates location of radial artery.
(From Wade JF: Comprehensive respiratory care, ed 3, St Louis, 1982, The CV Mosby Co.)

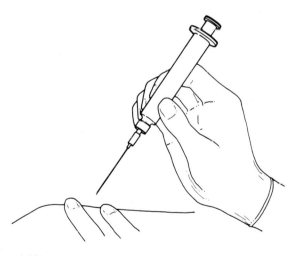

Figure 1-13
Technique for puncture of the radial artery. The syringe is held at its base and the finger of the free hand stabilizes the artery.
(From Wade JF: Comprehensive respiratory care, ed 3, St Louis, 1982, The CV Mosby Co.)

Table 1-7   Arterial blood gas data

Parameter	Normal	Acidosis	Alkalosis
pH	7.35-7.45	<7.35	>7.45
PaO_2	80-100 mm Hg	Normal	Normal
$PaCO_2$	35-45 mm Hg	Respiratory: >45	Respiratory: <35
		Metabolic: normal to decreased	Metabolic: normal to increased
HCO_3^-	22-26 mEq/L	Respiratory: normal to increased	Respiratory: normal to decreased
		Metabolic: decreased	Metabolic: increased

Table 1-8   Alterations in acid/base

Causes	Assessment Findings	Nursing Interventions
Respiratory Acidosis		
Hypoventilation	Decreased respiratory frequency (R_f)	Assess vital signs
Drug overdose	Serum CO_2 >26 mEq/L	Assess level of consciousness (LOC), note changes from baseline
Respiratory failure	pH <7.35	Elevate head of bed to facilitate ventilation/perfusion
Oversedation	$Paco_2$ >45	Provide cardiopulmonary resuscitation (CPR) if indicated
Cardiopulmonary arrest	Pao_2 normal or decreased	Prepare for intubation and/or mechanical ventilation
	Decreased LOC	Provide supplemental O_2
	Confusion	Assess lung sounds
	Headache, lethargy	Provide pulmonary hygiene
	Tachycardia, dysrhythmia, elevated serum potassium	
Respiratory Alkalosis		
Hyperventilation	Tachycardia	Assess vital signs
Inappropriate mechanical ventilation	LOC changes	Assess LOC changes from baseline
	Paraesthesia	Assess lung sounds

Continued.

Table 1-8   Alterations in acid/base—cont'd

Causes	Assessment Findings	Nursing Interventions
Head trauma	Tingling of extremities	Provide emotional support
Anxiety	pH >7.45	Reduce respiratory rate
Fever	Serum CO_2 <22 mEq/L or normal	
Congestive heart failure	Pao_2 normal or decreased	
Pulmonary embolism	Decreased serum potassium	
	Diaphoresis	
	Vertigo	
	Hyperactive reflexes	
Metabolic Acidosis	pH <7.35	
Diarrhea	Serum CO_2 <22 mEq/L	Assess vital signs
Ketoacidosis	$Paco_2$ <35	Assess LOC changes from baseline
Cardiopulmonary arrest	Pao_2 normal	Provide CPR if indicated
Renal failure	Elevated serum potassium	
Aspirin overdose	Headache	
Diabetes	Nausea	

Vomiting
Diarrhea
Convulsions
Tremors
Kussmaul's respirations

Assess vital signs
Assess LOC changes from baseline

Metabolic Alkalosis
Potent diuretics
Vomiting
Nasogastric (NG) suction
Alkali ingestion

pH >7.45
$Paco_2$ >45
Serum co_2 >26 mEq/L
Nausea
Vomiting
Diarrhea
Decreased serum potassium
Decreased serum chloride
Paraesthesias
Leg cramps

low the clinician to interpret the results accurately. Correct interpretation of the arterial blood gas results will allow the clinician to select the appropriate nursing interventions. Table 1-7 lists the parameters of arterial blood gas and alterations for acidosis and alkalosis. In Table 1-8 each of the four acid-base alterations is discussed, including causes, assessment findings, and suggested nursing interventions.

Minute Ventilation

Minute ventilation is the product of the respiratory rate and the tidal volume. Normal minute ventilation ($\dot{V}_E$) is 4 to 6 1/min. It reflects how efficiently carbon dioxide is removed from the body. Minute ventilations of greater than 10/min indicate a high work of breathing.

Diagnostic Tests
Pulmonary Function Tests (Table 1-9)

Pulmonary function testing is used to determine how well the respiratory system is working. Measurements include volume and flow rates of expired air and are made using a spirometer. Pulmonary function testing is used to diagnose obstructive and restrictive lung disease and as a screening test for measurement of disability (Fig. 1-14).

Obstructive disease is evidenced by:
    normal or decreased VC
    increased FRC
    increased TLC
    increased RV
    decreased $FEV_{1.0}$

Signs of restrictive disease include:
    decreased VC
    decreased FRC
    decreased TLC
    decreased RV
    normal or decreased $FEV_{1.0}$

Table 1-9 Pulmonary functions

Volumes/Capacity Measurement	How Measured	Clinical Significance
Tidal volume (V_T) Amount of air per breath	5-10 cc/kg Determined by spirometry	Decreased in restrictive disease
Vital capacity (VC) Complete exhalation following maximal inhalation	15 cc/kg includes V_T, IRV, and ERV Determined by spirometry	Decreased VC with decreased flow rates found in pulmonary edema, atelectasis, pulmonary congestion Decreased VC with normal or increased flow rates: head injury, drug overdose, pregnancy, ascites
Total lung capacity Total volume of lungs	Includes V_T, IRV, ERV, RV	Decreased: restrictive disease Increased: obstructive disease
Inspiratory capacity (IC) Largest amount of air inhaled after normal exhalation	V_T + IRV Determined by spirometry	Decreased in restrictive disease
Inspiratory Reserve Volume (IRV) Additional volume of air inspired after normal inspiration	IC − V_T	Not indicative of respiratory dysfunction
Functional Residual Capacity (FRC) Amount of air in lungs after normal exhalation	ERV + RV	Increased obstructive disease

Continued.

Table 1-9 Pulmonary functions—cont'd

Volumes/Capacity Measurement	How Measured	Clinical Significance
Expiratory Reserve Volume (ERV) Additional amount of air exhaled after normal exhalation	Determined by spirometry	Can vary with position; 25% of VC
Pulmonary Mechanics		
Forced Vital Capacity (FVC) Maximal exhalation following maximal inhalation	Determined by spirometry	Decreased FVC indicates resistance to expiratory flow as in bronchospasm, asthma, emphysema, or chronic bronchitis
Forced expiratory volume over 1 second (FEV_1)	75% to 80% of FVC measured by spirometry	Decrease indicates level of airway obstruction
Maximum voluntary ventilation (MVV)	Measured by spirometry	Decreased in obstructive and restrictive disease
Diffusing capacity for carbon dioxide	Calculated by comparing inhaled carbon dioxide to exhaled carbon dioxide	Decrease caused by thickening of alveolar capillary membranes, pulmonary fibrosis, interstitial pulmonary disease

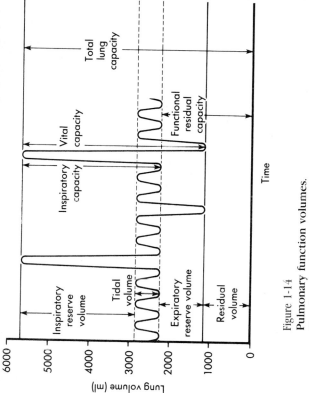

Figure 1-14
Pulmonary function volumes.
(From Perry A and Potter P: Shock, St Louis, 1983, The CV Mosby Co.)

Bronchoscopy

Bronchoscopy is the examination of the tracheobronchial tree to visualize the tree, obtain specimens such as sputum or biopsy, and retrieve foreign objects. A rigid or flexible bronchoscope may be used, with the flexible fiberoptic bronchoscope used most often. Major complications of bronchoscopy include regional hypoxia, hypoxemia, laryngospasm, bronchospasm, bleeding, or pneumothorax.

The nurse should monitor vital signs, respiratory status, and tracheobronchial secretions every 15 to 20 minutes following bronchoscopy until they are stable Table 1-10.

Thoracentesis

Thoracentesis is the removal of fluid from the pleural space. Excessive fluid can accumulate in the pleural space from direct insult to the thorax such as trauma or from an infection or disease. Diagnostic thoracentesis is performed to obtain samples of tissue or fluid to facilitate a differential diagnosis.

The nursing role during a thoracentesis includes positioning of the client (Fig. 1-15), assessment of vital signs, emotional support of the client, and evaluation of the client following the procedure (see box). The nurse must be alert for complications such as pneumothorax or inadvertent puncture of the lung or spleen during the procedure.

An important differentiation in assessing pleural fluid is exudate and transudate (Table 1-11). Exudates are pleural effusions caused by disease of the pleural membrane. Transudates are pleural effusions not associated with diseases of the pleural membrane (Waxman, 1989). Pleural fluid with a high protein level (>3 g/dl) and a specific gravity of 1.016 are considered exudates. Additional criteria include lactic dehydrogenase (LDH) of 200 Iv or greater, ratio of pleural fluid to serum protein of 0.5 or greater, ratio of pleural to serum LDH of 0.6 or greater, and a pleural red blood cell (RBC) count of 105 cells/mm^3 or greater (Light et al, 1972). Exudates are associated with neoplastic and inflammatory processes; transudates are associated with congestive heart failure, pulmonary and systemic hypertension, ascites, and cirrhosis.

Table 1-10 Nursing considerations following bronchoscopy

Nursing Action	Rationale
Vital Signs	
Monitor every 15-20 minutes until stable	Increased heart rate; respiratory rate may indicate hypoxia or bleeding
Sputum	
Monitor for increased production, color, consistency, bleeding	Increase in bloody sputum may indicate active bleeding post biopsy
Positioning	
Position client with head of bed elevated	Improves ventilation perfusion, helps reduce hypoxia
Client Education	
Restrict food and liquids until gag reflex returns; limit coughing, clearing of throat	Prevents aspiration
	Reduces possibility of dislodging clots, biopsy sites
No smoking	Irritation to mucosa
Hoarseness, sore throat	Expected temporarily following procedure

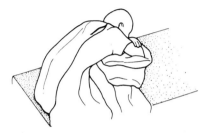

Figure 1-15
Position of client for thoracentesis.
(From Perry A and Potter P: Clinical nursing skills and techniques, ed 2, St Louis, 1990, The CV Mosby Co.)

Nursing Responsibilities During Thoracentesis

Assist client in positioning.
Provide reassurance.
Assess client's respiratory status.
Note characteristics of secretions aspirated.
Monitor vital signs.

Table 1-11   Pleural fluid assessment

Finding	Clinical Significance
Color	
Light/straw colored	Normal
Bloody	Hemothorax
	Trauma from procedure
	Tuberculosis
Purulent	Infectious process
	Emphysema
Cloudy/white	Inflammatory process
Laboratory Values	
Protein >3 g/dl	Neoplasm
	Tuberculosis
	Infection
<3 g/dl	CHF
	Ascites
	Systemic hypertension
	Pulmonary venous hypertension
Cell Count	
RBC = $10,000/mm^3$ pink/light red	Tissue damage
RBC >$10,000/mm^3$ grossly bloody	Intrapleural malignance
	Tuberculosis
	Chest trauma
	Hemothorax—**Note:** Hct of pleural fluid will be the same as venous blood
	CHF
	Cirrhosis
	Infection
	Pulmonary infarction
White blood cells (WBC) >$1,000/mm^3$	Pulmonary infection
	Tuberculosis
	Neoplasm
	Cirrhosis
	CHF
Neutrophils	Bacterial infection

Continued.

Table 1-11   Pleural fluid assessment—cont'd

Finding	Clinical Significance
Lymphocytes	
>50%	Tuberculosis
Blood clots	Neoplasm
	Tuberculosis
	Infection
Specific Gravity	
>1.016	Neoplasm
	Tuberculosis
	Infection
<1.104	CHF
Glucose	
Less than serum	Bacterial infection
	Inflammation
	Malignancies
	Tuberculosis
	Rheumatoid arthritis
Lactic Dehydrogenase (LDH)	
Elevated	Cancer
	Asbestosis
	Neoplasm
	Pulmonary infarction
	Infection
Decreased	Ascites
	CHF
	Hepatic cirrhosis
	Nephritis
Amylase	Pancreatitis
	Esophygeal rupture
Complement Levels	
Decreased	Rheumatoid arthritis
	Systemic lupus erythematosus
Elevated	Pyrogenic effusion
	Tuberculosis

Sputum Assessment

Much information regarding sputum production can be obtained from the client during the history. Sputum specimens are assessed for color, consistency, odor, and amount produced. Additionally, laboratory examination includes cultures and sensitivity, gram stain, and acid-fast stain. Sputum should be thin, white, and watery. Alterations in consistency are usually related to fluid volume depletion. Changes in color are associated with infection processes. Color may suggest the type of organisms causing the infection (Table 1-12).

Gram stain examination differentiates between gram negative and gram positive organisms. It also differentiates acute infection from colonization. Acute infectious processes have many white blood cells and are the probable bacterial cause of the infection. Colonized sputum has a mixture of organisms presenting with few WBCs indicating the lack of an acute problem. Acid-fast stain determines the presence of *Mycobacterium tuberculosis*. The culture and sensitivity tests provide a report of causative organisms and the susceptible antibiotics.

Radiographic Tests

Radiographic tests can provide much information about the clients' respiratory status. Table 1-13 lists the radiographic tests that are most frequently performed, the normal findings, and their clinical significance.

Table 1-12   Sputum assessment

Sputum Color	Possible Cause
Tan/pink	*Serratia*
Green	Chronic bronchitis
	Bronchiectasis
	Pseudomonas
	Acute bacterial
Yellow	Acute bacterial
Blood streaked	Mycoplasma
	Bronchitis
Rust	Old blood
	Tuberculosis

Table 1-13   Chest radiographic findings

Normal Findings	Alteration	Clinical Significance
Ribs		
12 to 8 attached; 4 floating	Widened intercostal spaces	Emphysema
Insert to sternum at 45° angle	Break	Air trapping
		Fracture
Mediastinum		
Space between the lungs	Deviation from side to side	Pulmonary fibrosis
		Tumor
		Pleural effusion
		Pneumothorax
	Widening	Neoplasms
		Aortic aneurysm
		Cor pulmonale
Trachea: midline; tubular	Deviation from midline	Tension pneumothorax
Translucent anterior mediastinum		Pleural effusion
		Atelectasis
		Mediastinal nodes
Heart	Width less than one half of the thorax	Hypertrophy
White, solid, anterior, left mediastinum		Cor pulmonale
Lung fields not visible	White, irregular patchy densities	Atelectasis
		Pneumonia

Normal findings	Abnormal findings	Causes
		Fibrosis
		Fluid
Hemidiaphragm rounded at base of thorax	Flattened	Chronic air trapping
		Emphysema
		Asthma
	Elevated	Active tuberculosis
		Pneumonia
		Phrenic nerve disease
		Pleurisy
		Pneumothorax
		Infection
Lung perfusion scan Uniform uptake of IV radiopharmaceutical; greater in dependent areas	Areas of low uptake	Poor perfusion
		Pneumonitis
Ventilation scan Equal gas distribution greater in apices	Unequal distribution	Poor ventilation
		Airway obstruction
Pulmonary angiography Even, unobstructed flow through pulmonary circulation	Interrupted blood flow	Emboli
		Stenosis
		Filling defects

Respiratory Monitoring

There are many ways to monitor both invasively and noninvasively various aspects of the respiratory system. Pulse oximetry provides noninvasive measures of arterial oxygen saturation (Table 1-14). The pulmonary artery catheter invasively measures pulmonary artery pressures, indirectly measures left heart function, and allows for measurement of the mixed venous bloods to determine oxygen transport and consumption.

Table 1-14   Pulse oximetry

Indications	Data	Nursing Considerations
Noninvasive arterial oxygen saturation monitoring (i.e., during weaning trials, after extubation, while weaning from oxygen therapy)	95%-100% <80%	Normal correlates with Pao_2 of 80-100 Decreased saturation, correlates with Pao_2 of ≤60 Indicates hypoxemia **Note:** Readings may be difficult to obtain in clients with peripheral vascular disease or those who smoke heavily or use nicotine gum

Pulmonary Artery Catheters

Invasive pulmonary artery (PA) catheters are capable of monitoring the pressure in the pulmonary artery: the pulmonary artery occlusive pressure and the right atrial pressure. By means of thermodilution, cardiac output can be determined. Continuous monitoring of $S_{\bar{v}}O_2$ can be accomplished with catheters containing fiberoptics. PA catheters are used in the care of critically ill clients to determine right-sided and left-sided heart function (Table 1-15).

Table 1-15 PA catheter measurements

Pressure	Reading	Significance
RA	2-6 mm Hg	Normal
	Decreased	Fluid volume depletion
	Elevated	Right ventricle (RV) failure
		Tamponade
		Pulmonary hypertension
		Chronic left ventricle (LV) failure
		Fluid volume overload
		Triscupid stenosis
		Constrictive pericarditis
PA	Systolic 20-30 mm Hg	Normal
	Diastolic <12 mm Hg	
	Mean <20 mm Hg	
	Decreased	Fluid volume depletion
	Increased	Pulmonary hypertension
		Mitral stenosis
		Chronic obstructive pulmonary disease (COPD)
		Left to right shunt
		LV failure

Continued.

Table 1-15   PA catheter measurements—cont'd

Pressure	Reading	Significance
PAWP	4-12 mm Hg	Reflects LA pressure
		Normal
	Decreased	Fluid volume depletion
	Elevation	LV failure
		Mitral stenosis
		Mitral insufficiency
		Constrictive pericarditis
		Volume overload
Cardiac output (CO)	4-6 l/min	Normal
Cardiac index (CI)	2.5-4.5 l/m/m^2	Normal
Mixed venous oxygen	36-42 tor	Normal
P$\overline{v}O_2$	>42 tor	Septic shock
		Excess inotrope administration
		Fever
		Poor sampling
		Left to right shunt

Saturation of venous oxygen $S\bar{v}O_2$		
	60%-80%	Normal
	>80%	Excessive FiO_2
		Wedged PA catheter
		Sepsis
		Anesthesia
		Hypothermia
	<60%	Hyperthermia
		Pain
		Shivering
		Anemia
		Seizures
		Inadequate FiO_2
		Shock
		Hypovolemia
		Suctioning
		Ventilator disconnect
		Positive expiratory end pressure (PEEP)
		Hemorrhage

References

Light RW, MacGregor I, and Luchsinger PC: Pleural effusions: the diagnostic separation of transudates and exudates, Ann Intern Med 77:507, 1972.

Malasanos L et al: Health assessment ed 14, St Louis, 1990, The CV Mosby Co.

Waxman K: Pleural disorders in Shoemaker, Ayres, Grenvik, Holbrook, and Thompson, Textbook of critical Care, ed 2, The Society of Critical Care Medicine, 1989, WB Saunders Co.

Bibliography

Ahrens TS: Concepts in the assessment of oxygenation, Focus on Critical Care 14(1)1:36-44 1987.

Ahrens TS and Rutherford KA: The new pulmonary math: applying the a/A ratio, Am J Nurs 87(3):337-340, 1987.

American Edwards Corporation: Understanding hemodynamic measurements made with the Swan-Ganz catheter, Am Edwards Laboratories, Santa Ana, Calif.

American Thoracic Society: Diagnostic standards and classification of tuberculosis and other mycobacterial diseases, American Review of Respiratory Disease 123(3), 1981.

Burns K and Johnson PJ: Health assessment in clinical practice, Englewood Cliffs, NJ, 1980, Prentice Hall, Prentice Hall Press.

Daily EK and Schroeder JS: Techniques in bedside hemodynamic monitoring, ed 4, St Louis, 1989, The CV Mosby Co.

Felson B, Weinstein AS, and Spitz HB: Principles of chest roentgenology: a programmed text, Philadelphia, 1965, WB Saunders Co.

Harper RW: A guide to respiratory care: physiology and clinical applications, Philadelphia, 1981, JB Lippincott Co.

Jacquith SM: The oximetrix opticath: What it is and how can it facilitate nursing management of the critically ill patient? Critical Care Nurse, May/June: 55-58, 1984.

Loudon R and Murphy R: State of the art: Lung sounds. American Review of Respiratory Disease, 130:663-673, 1984.

Nellcor Incorporated: Hemoglobin and the principles of pulse eximetry, Reference note number 1, Nellcor Incorporated, 1987, Calif.

Nellcor Incorporated: Principles of pulse oximetry, Nellcor Incorporated, 1988, Calif.

Palmer PN: Advanced hemodynamic assessment: Dimensions of Critical Care Nursing 1(3):139-144, 1982.

Perry AG and Potter PA: Clinical nursing skills and techniques, ed 2, St Louis 1989, The CV Mosby Co.

Seidel HM et al: Mosby's guide to physical examination, St Louis, 1987, The CV Mosby Co.

Shapiro BA, Harrison RA, and Trout CA: Clinical application of respiratory care, ed 3, Chicago, 1982, Year Book Medical Publishers, Inc.

Waxman K: Pleural disorders in Shoemaker, Ayres, Grenvik, Holbrook, and Thompson, Textbook of Critical Care, ed 2, The Society of Critical Care Medicine, 1989, WB Saunders Co.

Wilkins RL, Hodgkin JE, and Lopez B: Lung sounds: a practical guide, St Louis, 1988, The CV Mosby Co.

Wyngaarden JB and Smith LH: Cecil textbook of medicine, vol 1, ed 18, 1988, WB Saunders Co.

Nursing Diagnosis

Nursing diagnosis is defined as "a clinical judgment about an individual, family, or community that is derived through a deliberate, systematic process of data collection and analysis. It provides the basis for prescriptions for definitive therapy for which the nurse is accountable. It is expressed concisely and it includes the etiology of the condition when known" (Shoemaker, 1984). A nursing diagnosis is comprised of the client's problem, a "related to" statement defining the etiology, and the clinical signs and symptoms specific to the problem (Kim, 1987). Clustering of data assessed during physical assessment and review of diagnostic test results will assist the nurse in selecting the appropriate nursing diagnoses for the client.

Reviewing all available data before selecting a diagnosis is important. Too often nursing diagnoses are selected based on the medical plan of care rather than the nursing care needs. The approved nursing diagnoses as defined by the North American Nursing Diagnoses Association (NANDA) includes a definition of the diagnosis, the related factors, and the defining characteristics. The nurse should review all the defining characteristics for each diagnosis, selecting the one that describes the client's nursing care needs. The plan of care can then be developed to achieve the expected outcomes for the client. Expected outcomes are measures of the success or progress of the nursing interventions. Since these expected outcomes are client centered and measureable, the nurse is able to document and measure client progress systematically.

NANDA defines three respiratory nursing diagnoses: ineffective airway clearance, ineffective breathing pattern, and impaired gas exchange.

Ineffective Airway Clearance

Definition: The state in which an individual is unable to clear secretions or obstructions from the respiratory tract to maintain airway patency.

Related Factors:
Decreased energy and fatigue
Tracheobronchial infection, obstruction, or secretion
Perceptual and/or cognitive impairment

Defining Characteristics:
Abnormal breath sounds: crackles, wheezes, rhonchus
Changes in respiratory rate or depth
Tachypnea (increased respiratory rate)
Cough, effective/ineffective, with or without sputum
Cyanosis
Dyspnea, at rest or on exertion
Fever

Ineffective Breathing Pattern

Definition: The state in which an individual's inhalation and/or exhalation pattern does not enable adequate ventilation.

Related Factors:
Neuromuscular impairment
Pain
Musculoskeletal impairment
Perceptual or cognitive impairment
Anxiety
Decreased energy and fatigue
Inflammatory process
Decreased lung expansion
Tracheobronchial obstruction

Defining Characteristics:
Dyspnea
Shortness of breath
Tachypnea
Fremitus
Abnormal arterial blood gases
Cyanosis
Cough
Nasal flaring

Respiratory depth changes
Assumption of three-point position; orthopeanic position
Pursed lip breathing; prolonged expiratory phase
Increased anteroposterior diameter
Use of accessory muscles
Altered chest expansion

Impaired Gas Exchange

Definition: The state in which the individual experiences an imbalance between oxygen uptake and carbon dioxide elimination at the alveolar-capillary gas exchange area.

Related Factors:

Altered oxygen supply
Alveolar-capillary membrane changes
Altered blood flow
Altered oxygen-carrying capacity of blood

Defining Characteristics:

Confusion
Somnolence
Irritability
Inability to move secretions
Hypercapnea
Hypoxia

Related Nursing Diagnoses

The following nursing diagnoses are nursing care problems frequently associated with clients with respiratory alterations.

Activity Intolerance

A state in which an individual has insufficient physiologic or psychologic energy to endure or complete required or desired daily activities.

Related Factors	Defining Characteristics
Generalized weakness	Verbal report of fatigue or weakness
Sedentary life-style	
Imbalance between oxygen supply and demand	Abnormal heart rate or blood pressure response to activity
Bedrest	Exertional discomfort or dyspnea
Immobility	
	ECG changes reflecting arrhythmias or ischemia

Ineffective Individual Coping

Impairment of adaptive behaviors and problem-solving abilities of a person in meeting life's demands and roles.

Related Factors	Defining Characteristics
Situational crisis	Verbalization of inability to cope or inability to ask for help
Maturational crisis	
Personal vulnerability	Inability to meet role expectations
Multiple life changes	Inability to problem solve
No vacations	Alteration in societal participation
Inadequate relaxation	Destructive behavior toward self or others
Inadequate support systems	
Little or no exercise	Inappropriate use of defense mechanisms
Poor nutrition	Change in usual communication patterns
Unmet expectations	
	Verbal manipulation
	High illness rate
	High rate of accidents
	Overeating
Work overload	Lack of appetite
Too many deadlines	Excessive smoking
Unrealistic perceptions	Excessive drinking
	Overuse of prescribed tranquilizers
	Alcohol

Related Factors	Defining Characteristics
	Chronic fatigue
	Insomnia
	Muscular tension
	Ulcers
	Frequent headaches
	Frequent neckaches
	Irritable bowel
	Chronic worry
	General irritability
	Poor self-esteem
	Chronic anxiety
	Emotional tension
	Chronic depression

Knowledge Deficit (Specify)

A state in which specific information is lacking.

Related Factors	Defining Characteristics
Lack of exposure	Verbalization of the problem
Lack of recall	Inaccurate follow-through of instruction
Information misinterpretation	
Cognitive limitation	Inadequate performance of test
Lack of interest in learning	Inappropriate or exaggerated behaviors: anger, hostility, apathy, hysteria
Unfamiliarity with information resources	
	Statement of misconception
Client's request for no information	Request for information

Altered Nutrition: Less than Body Requirements

The state in which an individual experiences an intake of nutrients insufficient to meet metabolic needs.

Related Factors	Defining Characteristics
Inability to ingest food, digest food, or absorb nutrients because of biologic, psychologic, or economic factors	Loss of weight with adequate food intake
	Body weight 20% or more under ideal for height and frame
	Reported inadequate food intake less than recommended daily allowances (RDA)
	Weakness of muscles required for swallowing or mastication
	Reported evidence of lack of food
	Lack of interest in food
	Perceived inability to ingest food
	Aversion to eating
	Reported altered taste sensation
	Satiety immediately after ingesting food
	Abdominal pain with or without pathologic conditions
	Sore, inflamed buccal cavity

Altered Health Maintenance

Inability to identify, manage, or seek help to maintain health.

Related Factors	Defining Characteristics
Lack of or significant alteration in communication skills	Demonstrated lack of knowledge regarding basic health practices
Inability to make deliberate and thoughtful judgments	
Perceptual or cognitive impairment	Demonstrated lack of adaptive behaviors to internal or external environmental changes
Alteration in fine and/or gross motor skills	

Related Factors	Defining Characteristics
Ineffective individual coping	Reported or observed inability to take responsibility for meeting basic health practices in any or all functional pattern areas
Dysfunctional grieving	
Lack of material resources	
Unachieved developmental tasks	
	History of lack of health-seeking behavior
Ineffective family coping	
Disabling spiritual distress	Reported or observed lack of equipment and financial or other resources
	Reported or observed impairment of personal support system

CASE STUDY
History of Present Illness

A 24-year-old unemployed woman comes to the emergency room with complaints of "can't breathe." Her severe shortness of breath started during the night and has progressively worsened. She has been treated for asthma for 16 years, requiring frequent hospital admissions and a complex medical regimen. Current medications include a 24-hour sustained action oral theophylline, a beta-agonist–metered dose inhaler 4 times per day, and a steroid–metered-dose inhaler 4 times a day. She completed a course of tapering oral steroids 10 days ago. Current complaints include extreme shortness of breath, severe nonproductive cough, tightening chest, increasing fatigue, and a feeling of impending doom. Compliance with her medication regimen is questionable. She last took her metered-dose inhaler before coming to the emergency room. She cannot remember when she last took her other medications. She denies recent fever, chills, night sweats, change in sputum color or character, or pedal edema.

Past Medical History

Illnesses:	Frequent hospital admissions for exacerbation of asthma; three admissions in past 4 months requiring oral steroids and hospitalization
Familial:	Noncontributing
Pets:	Two cats, one dog
Marital status:	Divorced

Children: Two boys, ages 2 and 4
Social
  history: Lives with mother and grandmother in four-room
               apartment on the tenth floor of a high-rise apart-
               ment building. No air conditioning is available.
               She is currently unemployed because of her fre-
               quent illnesses and hospitalizations.
Allergies: Dust, pollen, aspirin, sulfa drugs, pet dander
Smoking: One to two packs/day; 20-pack year history
Alcoholic
  use: One to two beers/day

Review of Systems:

General: The client is an obese female who appears older
              than her stated age. She is alert and oriented, sit-
              ting in the orthopneaic position using accessory
              muscles of respiration and using pursed lip
              breathing; has prolonged expiration. She is dia-
              phoretic and anxious.
Vital signs: Temperature 38° C
              Pulse 136/min
              Respiration 32/min
              Blood pressure 168/94
              Paradoxial pulse of 18 mm Hg
              Height: 5'2" Weight: 246 lbs
HEENT: Nasal flaring with inspiration
              Oral mucosa is dusky
              Normocephalic
              No oral lesions noted
Neck: Full range of motion
              Trachea midline
              No stridor
              Mild jugular venous distension with respiration
              No cervical or supraclavicular lymphadenopathy
              Carotid pulses 2+; no bruits
Chest: Increased AP diameter
              Decreased expansion with respiration
              Hyperresonant to percussion
              Sternal and intracostal retraction
Heart: Slightly irregular; 136 beats/min; no murmurs,
              gallops, or rubs
Lungs: Diffuse expiratory wheezing; prolonged expira-
              tory phase through pursed lips.

Abdomen:	Nontender to palpation. Exam difficult to perform because of client's inability to recline
Extremities:	Slight ankle edema
	Pulses 2+ and symmetric
Activity:	No regular exercise; self-care adequate
Reproductive:	LMP 7/11/90. Pap smear: unknown
Sleep:	8 to 10 hours per night, requires occasional sleeping pill
Neurologic:	Alert, oriented. Reflexes intact
Gastrointestinal (GI):	Bowel movement daily. No c/o with urination; normal bowel sounds

Laboratory Data

Pulmonary function:	FEV_1 1.0 liter
	FVC 3.5 liters
ABG:	pH 7.35/$Paco_2$ 45/PaO_2 40
CBC:	WBC 13,000/mm^3
	Hgb 13 g%
	Hct 40%
	Seqs 75%
	Band 5%
	Lymphs 20%
Chest radiography:	Anterior pulmonary hyperexpansion. Cardiac silhouette and pulmonary vasculature are relatively normal. Lateral film shows a flattened diaphragm.

Nursing Care Plan

Diagnosis	Expected Outcome	Nursing Intervention
Ineffective breathing pattern related to respiratory muscle fatigue/ impaired respiratory mechanics	Client will pace activities to minimize respiratory muscle fatigue as evidenced by reported decrease in dyspnea, reduced respiratory rate, and average tidal volume	Teach client pursed lip breathing, diaphragmatic breathing, and controlled cough techniques. Teach client energy-conserving techniques, e.g., stair climbing, bed making, and lifting.

Diagnosis	Expected Outcome	Nursing Intervention
		Monitor breathing pattern, and assess for effectiveness every 2 hours.
		Monitor general appearance for color, respiratory rate, and depth and mental status every 2 hours.
		Initiate referral for pulmonary clinical nurse specialist.
	Client will use relaxation techniques for breathing control as evidence by reported decrease in episodes of shortness of breath	Teach client progressive relaxation techniques.
Impaired gas exchange related to alveolar hypoventilation	Client achieves optimal respiratory function without evidence of hypoxemia	Review ABG results and correlate with clinical condition.
		Institute measures to improve airway clearance, e.g., encourage 3 to 5 liters of fluids by mouth per day.
		Provide supplemental oxygen during activity/sleep per physician order.

Diagnosis	Expected Outcome	Nursing Intervention
		Maintain airway patency.
		Pace and schedule activity to reduce oxygen demands
		Position client to facilitate adequate ventilation/ perfusion.
Lack of knowledge (asthma and treatment) related to lack of recall	Client will verbalize knowledge of implications of health practices	Discuss health practices with client.
	Client will be able to state causative factors for asthma	Assist client with identification of causative factors.
		Teach client identification of respiratory irritants and ways to avoid exposure.
		Teach client pulmonary hygiene measures, pursed lip breathing, and controlled cough technique.
		Review medications, including dosage, administration, frequency, and side effects.
		Teach client to monitor color, consistency, and amount of sputum.

References

Kim MJ, McFarland GK, and McLane AM: Pocket guide to nursing diagnoses, ed 3, St Louis, 1989, The CV Mosby Co.

Shoemaker JK: Essential features of a nursing diagnosis. In Kim MJ, McFarland GK, and McLane AM, editors, Classification of Nursing Diagnoses. Proceedings of the Fifth National Conference, St Louis, 1984, The CV Mosby Co.

Bibliography

Gordon M: Manual of nursing diagnosis 1984-1985, St Louis, 1986, McGraw-Hill, Inc.

Hanley MV and Tyler ML: Ineffective airway clearance related to airway infection, Nurs Clin North Am 22(1), 1987.

Kim MJ and Larson JL: Ineffective airway clearance and ineffective breathing patterns: theoretical and research base for nursing diagnosis, Nurs Clin North Am 22(1), 1987.

Respiratory Alterations

3

Acute Alterations
Acute Respiratory Failure

Acute respiratory failure (ARF) is the result of inadequate gas exchange in the lungs. It can be defined as an arterial oxygen partial pressure of less than 50 mm Hg and/or a carbon dioxide partial pressure of greater than 50 mm Hg. ARF is associated with impairment of ventilation perfusion matching, respiratory muscle fatigue, impaired ventilatory drive, and hemodynamic alterations (Petty, 1989).

Assessment Data	Nursing Interventions	Special Considerations
Dyspnea at rest	Assess vital signs	May require intubation and mechanical ventilation
Anxiety	Elevate the head of bed 30-45 degrees	
Tachypnea		
Tachycardia		Continuous pulse oximetry may be helpful in monitoring oxygenation
Confusion	Note respiratory pattern	
$Pao_2 < 50$ mm Hg	Assist/instruct client in controlled breathing exercises, e.g., pursed lip breathing	
$Paco_2 > 50$ mm Hg		
Slightly elevated blood pressure		
Cyanosis may be evident		
	Reassure client that he or she will not be alone during episodes of respiratory distress	

Assessment Data	Nursing Interventions	Special Considerations
	Supplemental oxygen therapy may be indicated	
	Monitor effectiveness of oxygen therapy	

Adult Respiratory Distress Syndrome

Adult respiratory distress syndrome (ARDS) is a multi-symptomed syndrome manifested by hypoxemia, decreased lung compliance, diffuse alveolar infiltrates on x-ray examination, and respiratory failure requiring mechanical ventilation. Other names for ARDS include shock lung, wet lung, posttraumatic pulmonary insufficiency, obliterative alveolitis, hyaline lung, noncardiogenic pulmonary edema, post pump lung, and Da Nang lung. ARDS can be caused by trauma, sepsis, pulmonary or fat emboli, oxygen toxicity, shock, near drowning, or fluid volume overload, as well as other conditions.

Assessment Data	Nursing Interventions	Special Considerations
Agitation	Maintain airway patency	Usually requires intubation and mechanical ventilation
Hyperventilation	Assess lung sounds	
Cyanosis	Assess vital signs	
Tachypnea	Monitor respiratory rate, pattern	Multi-system failure requires frequent monitoring of all body systems
Increased tracheobronchial secretions	Elevate head of bed 30-45 degrees	
Crackles	Monitor oxygenation via oximetry or ABGs as required	Plan nursing care measures to reduce oxygen demands
Rhonchi		
Hypotension		
Hypoxemia: Pao_2 < 55% on room air		Client is usually transferred to intensive care unit

Assessment Data	Nursing Interventions	Special Considerations
$Sao_2 < 85\%$ on supplemental oxygen		May require cardiac monitoring for arrhythmias secondary to tissue hypoxia
		Anticipate the need of invasive hemodynamic monitoring as a diagnostic tool to determine fluid status

Acute Bronchitis

Acute bronchitis is an acute inflammation of the bronchial mucous membrane of the tracheobronchial tree usually as a complication of or associated with other pulmonary diseases. It is predominantly caused by viral or bacterial organisms.

Assessment Data	Nursing Interventions	Special Considerations
Chest tightness	Assess vital signs	Chest physiotherapy may be indicated if the client cannot effectively mobilize sputum
Fever	Assess lung sounds	
Chills	Encourage oral fluid intake of 1-2 L/ day if not contraindicated by cardiovascular status	
Cough		
Wheezing		Supplemental oxygen may be needed if hypoxemia develops
Rhonchi		
Sputum production 30 cc/24 hr		
Shortness of breath	Encourage deep breathing and coughing	
	Encourage activity within the client's limits	

Assessment Data	Nursing Interventions	Special Considerations
	Bronchodilators are indicated for the relief of bronchospasm and decreasing airway resistance	

Chronic Alterations
Chronic Obstructive Pulmonary Disease

Chronic obstructive pulmonary disease (COPD) is characterized by airway obstruction and decreased expiratory flow. Emphysema, chronic bronchitis, asthma, and bronchiectasis are the most common forms of COPD. The two components thought to be reversible in COPD are airway diameter and expiratory flow rates, which can be manipulated through the use of bronchodilators and pulmonary hygiene therapies. Clients with chronically elevated carbon dioxide levels above 45 mm Hg are stimulated to breathe by changes in their oxygen levels rather than by a rising $Paco_2$. Administration of oxygen at levels usually greater than 3 L/min may suppress the hypoxic drive to breathe in these individuals. Therefore, clients with chronic CO_2 retention are at increased risk to develop respiratory depression when oxygen therapy is administered. It is important to note that all clients with the diagnosis of COPD are not CO_2 retainers.

Chronic Bronchitis

Chronic bronchitis is an inflammation of the tracheobronchial tree characterized by fibrotic and atropic changes in the bronchial mucous membrane. It occurs frequently among clients who smoke and in some individuals with asthma.

Assessment Data	Nursing Interventions	Special Considerations
Persistent cough	Instruct client to be aware of the signs of acute infections (fever, chills, sputum change)	Recommend community-based pulmonary rehabilitation program if appropriate
Dyspnea on exertion		
Purulent sputum		
Unexplained weight gain		
Cyanosis	Instruct client in pursed lip breathing techniques to decrease sensation of dyspnea	Administer oxygen therapy cautiously in clients who retain carbon dioxide
Crackles		
Rhonchi		
Cor pulmonale		
Tachycardia	Instruct client in fluid intake of 1-2 L/day unless contraindicated by cardiovascular status	
Dyspnea at rest		
Pedal edema		
Crackles in the base of the lung		
Elevated hemoglobin	Instruct client in proper handling of respiratory secretions	
Abnormal pulmonary function test: Decreased vital capacity; increased functional residual capacity; decreased FEV_1; increased total lung capacity	Monitor supplemental oxygen if ordered	
Abnormal arterial blood gas: Decreased Pao_2; normal or elevated $Paco_2$		

Emphysema

Emphysema is characterized by the progressive destruction of alveolar sacs and the supporting structures. Physical signs include the classic barrel chest with use of accessory muscles of respiration in the advanced stages. Clients with the diagnosis of emphysema often have a history of smoking. Emphysema does occur as a result of alph$_1$ antitrypsin deficiency.

Assessment Data	Nursing Interventions	Special Considerations
Dyspnea on exertion and at rest	Instruct client in diaphragmatic and pursed lip breathing	Recommend community-based pulmonary rehabilitation program if appropriate
Decreased weight		
Chronic cough with little sputum production	Instruct client in energy conservation techniques	Not all clients with emphysema chronically retain CO_2
Barrel chest		
Use of accessory muscles of respiration	Promote compliance with medication regimen	Lung sounds may be markedly reduced because of decreased air movement and air trapping
Digital clubbing	Encourage participation in a regular exercise program as indicated	
Peripheral or central cyanosis		
Hyperresonant to percussion	Provide nutritional information and dietary consultation as indicated to promote adequate nutrition	Avoid use of sedatives and tranquilizers since they may depress respirations
Crackles		
Wheezes		
Elevated hemoglobin		
Abnormal pulmonary function test: Decreased vital capacity; increased total lung capacity; Increased functional residual capacity; decreased $FEV_{1.0}$		

Asthma

Typically asthma is a narrowing of the airways as a result of inflammation and edema of the mucosal wall associated with excessive sputum production and wheezing. The process can be triggered by allergens or irritants such as odors, weather, and stress.

Assessment Data	Nursing Interventions	Special Considerations
Acute Phase		
Anxiety	Assess and monitor vital signs frequently	Observe closely for fatigue
Dyspnea		
Use of accessory muscles of respiration	Encourage use of controlled breathing	May require intubation and mechanical ventilation if work of breathing is excessive
Chest hyperinflation	Position with head of bed elevated 45-90 degrees	
Diaphoresis		Be alert for a rising $Paco_2$ with tachypnea and respiratory distress
Tachycardia		
Hypertension	Provide nebulized bronchodilators as indicated	
Wheezing		
Pulsus paradoxus	Provide supplemental oxygen as indicated	
Decreased Pao_2		
Rising $Paco_2$		
Falling pH	Provide hydration by oral route if appropriate or intravenously if indicated	
Decreased $FEV_{1.0}$		
Increased residual volume		
Increased total lung capacity	Monitor oxygenation via pulse oximetry or ABGs as appropriate	

Assessment Data	Nursing Interventions	Special Considerations
Chronic Phase		
Asymptomatic or mild dyspnea on exertion	Assess predisposing factors for asthma	
	Instruct client in medication regime including dosage, frequency, and side effects	
	Instruct in use of over-the-counter medications	
	Instruct in proper use of metered-dose inhalers	.

Restrictive Disease

Lung disease that results in impaired inhalation and restriction to lung expansion is defined as restrictive. Restrictive may be caused by interstitial lung disease (such as pulmonary fibrosis) or extrapulmonary, as in obesity, pregnancy, and musculoskeletal deformities. Diminished lung compliance increases the client's work of breathing. Typically the total lung capacity and the vital capacity are reduced.

Interstitial Pulmonary Fibrosis

Interstitial pulmonary fibrosis is a diffuse inflammatory process resulting in cellular thickening of the alveolar walls and a decrease in lung compliance.

Assessment Data	Nursing Interventions	Special Considerations
Progressive dyspnea	Assess vital signs	May benefit from pulmonary rehabilitation to assist with modification of activities of daily living
Digital clubbing	Monitor respiratory pattern for rate	
Tachypnea		
Cyanosis	Monitor serial ABGs	
Cough		
Diffuse crepitations	Steroid therapy may be indicated	
Exercise hypoxia	Oxygen therapy may be indicated	
Decreased vital capacity		
	Teach factors to prevent infection	

Sarcoidosis

Sarcoidosis is a granulomatous disease involving many systems. It is manifested by lymphadenopathy; pulmonary infiltrates; and skeletal, skin, liver, and eye lesions. It occurs most frequently in young adults between the ages of 20 to 40 years and more often in young black females. Sarcoidosis can occur as an acute process, which usually resolves within a 2-year period, or as a chronic, progressive disease with progressive pulmonary disability (Springhouse 1989a).

Assessment Data	Nursing Interventions	Special Considerations
Positive Kuem-Siltzbach test	Assess vital signs	A pulmonary rehabilitation program may be beneficial
Malaise	Assess respiratory status	
Arthralgia	Provide analgesics for arthralgia	
Cough		
Erythema nodosum	Encourage fluid intake	
Paratracheal adenopathy by chest radiography	Monitor weight	
Fatigue	Monitor for adverse effects of steroids	

Assessment Data	Nursing Interventions	Special Considerations
Decreased PaO_2	Instruct client in importance of following medical regimen	
Hypercalcemia		
Decreased diffusing capacity as measured by pulmonary function testing		

Pleural Effusion

Pleural effusions are the result of excessive accumulation of fluid in the pleural space and have many causes. The fluid that collects is categorized as a transudative (low protein fluid) or exudative (high protein fluid).

Transudative effusion is characterized by ascites, systemic hypertension, pulmonary hypertension, CHF, hepatic cirrhosis, and nephritis. Exudative effusion is characterized by pulmonary infarctions and neoplasms.

Assessment Data	Nursing Interventions	Special Considerations
Dyspnea	Assess vital signs	Prepare for possible thoracentesis
Chest pain	Assess respiratory rate, pattern, and chest wall movement	
Cough		
Splinting on respiration		
Dullness to percussion	Provide emotional support during periods of dyspnea and during the thoracentesis	
Absent or decreased lung sounds over the affected area		
Hypoxemia	Assess lung sounds	
S_3 gallop	Position in semi-Fowler's for comfort and to facilitate adequate ventilation	
Decreased tidal volume		

Obesity Hypoventilation Syndrome (Pickwickian Syndrome)

Obesity hypoventilation syndrome is caused by excessive weight on the thorax resulting in restriction to chest wall movement and hypoventilation. Generally clients in excess of 300 to 400 pounds will have restriction to chest wall movement and may not be able to lie supine without feeling short of breath.

Assessment Data	Nursing Interventions	Special Considerations
Morbid obesity	Instruct client regarding the relationship between weight and breathlessness	May develop respiratory failure resulting in need for intubation and mechanical ventilation
Hypersomnolence		
Elevated $PaCO_2$		
Decreased Pa_{O_2}		
Irregular sleep pattern	Instruct client in weight reduction diet	May have sleep apnea
	Instruct client regarding consequences of	

Infections
Pneumonia

Pneumonia is an acute infection of the lung parenchyma, which may lead to impaired gas exchange. Pneumonias can be caused by bacterial, fungal, or viral infections. Additionally, aspiration of foreign substance can result in pneumonia.

Viral pneumonias begin with cold or flu-like symptoms. The infection progresses to high fever, productive cough, and may result in respiratory failure. Bacterial pneumonias are frequent complications of viral pneumonias.

Assessment Data	Nursing Interventions	Special Considerations
Influenza		
Cough	Assess vital signs	May require intubation and mechanical ventilation
Purulent sputum	Maintain adequate fluid intake	
Sudden chills		
Febrile	Elevate head of bed 45 degrees	Bacterial pneumonia is a frequent complication seen in the elderly population
Crackles	Assess respirations and lung sounds	
Dyspnea		
Headache	Administer antibiotics and antipyretics if required	
Chestwall pain		
Adenovirus		
Fever	Assess vital signs	Low mortality
Chills	Assess respiratory pattern	Frequently observed in young adults
Sore throat		
Cough	Provide symptom management, e.g., antipyretics, antibiotics as needed	
Rhinitis		
Chest pain		
Crackles		
Few rhonchus		
Malaise		
Lymphadenopathy		
Patchy pneumonia on x-ray examination		
WBC slightly elevated		

Assessment Data	Nursing Interventions	Special Considerations
Cytomegalovirus (CMV)		
Fever of unknown origin	Assess vital signs	Associated with immunosuppressed clients
Malaise	Assess respiratory pattern	
Lymphadenopathy	Provide protective isolation for immunosuppressed clients	May require intubation and mechanical ventilation
Enlarged liver		
Enlarged spleen		
Cough	Elevate head of bed	
Shaking chills	Provide and monitor supplemental oxygen as indicated	
Dyspnea		
Crackles		
Cyanosis		
Patchy infiltrates on chest x-ray examination		
Pneumocystitis Carinii (PCP)		
Fever	Assess vital signs	Most commonly seen in clients with acquired immune deficiency syndrome (AIDS)
Shortness of breath	Assess respiratory status for rate and pattern	
Dry, nonproductive cough	Supplemental oxygen may be required	
Hypoxia		May require intubation and mechanical ventilation
Chills	Assess and monitor hypoxemia by ABGs or pulse oximetry as indicated	
Malaise		May need protective isolation for client who is immunosuppressed

Assessment Data	Nursing Interventions	Special Considerations
	Plan nursing care activities to reduce oxygen demands	
	Provide frequent rest periods	
	Monitor effects of oxygen therapy by ABGs or pulse oximetry as indicated	

Bacterial Pneumonia

Pneumonia caused by bacteria that results in alveolar inflammation is bacterial pneumonia. Atelectasis is a common finding resulting from exudate in the alveoli.

Assessment Data	Nursing Interventions	Special Considerations
Staphylococcus		
Dyspnea	Assess vital signs	May need chest tube placement for empyema
Sudden chills	Provide adequate hydration	
Fever 38.9-40.0° C		Oxicillin resistant *Staphylococcus aureus* is very resistant to therapy and requires isolation
Blood-tinged sputum	Elevate head of bed 45 degrees	
Tachycardia	Monitor respiratory pattern, rate	
Elevated WBC	Administer antibiotic therapy as indicated to maintain therapeutic blood level	
Infiltrates on chest X-ray examination		
	Provide supplemental oxygen as indicated	

Assessment Data	Nursing Interventions	Special Considerations
Klebsiella		
Fever	Assess vital signs	Frequently seen in debilitated clients or clients with chronic illness
Chills	Assess respiratory status: rate, pattern	
Productive cough		
Cyanosis	Supplemental oxygen may be required	
Shallow respirations		
Upper lobe consolidation	Encourage fluid intake by mouth of 1-2 L/day	
Elevated WBC		
	Monitor sputum production for amount, color, consistency	
Streptococcus		
Sudden onset of symptoms	Assess vital signs	
Fever 38.9-40.0° C	Assess respiratory pattern, rate	
Productive cough	Monitor sputum for color, amount, consistency	
Thick yellow/green sputum		
Elevated WBC	Provide chest physiotherapy as indicated	
Lobar consolidation		
Frequently preceded by an upper respiratory infection	Encourage fluid intake by mouth of 1-2 L/day	

Assessment Data	Nursing Interventions	Special Considerations
Legionella Pneumophila (Legionnaire's Disease)		
Anorexia	Assess vital signs	May require intubation and mechanical ventilation
Malaise	Assess respiratory pattern	
Generalized weakness	Supplemental oxygen may be indicated	Provide a safe environment for the client due to periods of confusion
Chills		
Fever of sudden onset and rapid rise	Reorient to place, person, time frequently	Plan of nursing care may need to be altered to reduce oxygen demands and consumption
Cough	Provide symptomatic relief for fever and discomfort	
Nausea		
Vomiting		
Pleuritic chest pain	Provide emotional support especially during periods of confusion and disorientation	
Confusion		
Dyspnea		
Tachypnea		
Bradycardia		
Patchy infiltrates on chest x-ray examination	Monitor sputum production for amount, color, and consistency	
Pleural effusion	Monitor oxygen therapy with ABGs or pulse oximetry as appropriate	
Elevated WBC		

Aspiration Pneumonia

The introduction of a foreign substance into the lung, such as gastric contents, tube feeding, or fluids, can result in the development of aspiration pneumonia. It is found frequently in clients with chronic alcoholism, postcardiopulmonary arrest, or vomiting and in clients with poor or absent gag reflexes or decreased levels of consciousness.

Assessment Data	Nursing Interventions	Special Considerations
Decreased breath sounds	Assess vital signs	Clients intubated with endotracheal or tracheostomy tubes are at increased risk of aspiration pneumonia
Foul-smelling secretions	Assess respiratory rate and pattern	
Sputum may resemble vomitus	Monitor for further aspiration by testing tracheal aspirate for glucose content with a Dextrostix	
Elevated WBC		Clients are at risk of developing ARDS
Fever		
Decreased $Paco_2$	Suction tracheobronchially to help remove any aspirated material	Elderly clients may not exhibit the increased heart rate and respiratory rate
Decreased Pao_2		
Decreased Sao_2		
Tachypnea		
Tachycardia		

Tuberculosis

Tuberculosis (TB) is caused by infection with *Mycobacterium tuberculosis*. It can be acute or chronic and is most often seen in populations living in close quarters and those with little or no health care or prevention. Because of the number of immunosuppressed clients, the AIDS epidemic, and the increased exposure of health care workers to these clients, the incidence of tuberculosis is on the rise.

Assessment Data	Nursing Interventions	Special Considerations
Positive sputum for acid-fast bacilli	Assess vital signs	Incubation period is 4-8 weeks
Fatigue	Monitor sputum production especially for hemoptysis	Clients may be asymptomatic during the infectious stages
Weakness		
Night sweats		
Weight loss	Provide isolation as ordered	
Low grade fever	Instruct client and family on transmission sources	
Purulent sputum		

Assessment Data	Nursing Interventions	Special Considerations
Hemoptysis		Client should be isolated under respiratory precautions if suspicious symptoms are present
Lung consolidation	Instruct client and family on importance of following medical/nursing plan of care and need for followup	
Crackles		
Wheezes		
Upper lobe patchy infiltrates		Medications used to treat TB can cause peripheral neuritis or lead to hepatitis
Cavitation		
	Instruct client contacts to obtain skin testing	
	Instruct client to eat well-balanced diet. If anorexic, offer small, frequent feedings.	
	Promote rest by planning nursing care and procedures to allow for rest	

Lung Cancer

Lung cancer is the nation's most serious cancer problem (Groenwald, 1987). Lung cancer is caused by repeated irritation of lung mucosa by cigarette smoke, pollution, and occupational exposure. Lung cancer survival rates at 5 years are about 10% (Groenwald, 1987).

Assessment Data	Nursing Interventions	Special Considerations
Nonsmall Cell		
Epidermoid/Squamous Cell		
Cough Hoarseness Dyspnea Chest pain Wheezing	Provide pain management Provide preoperative teaching regarding deep breathing and coughing Provide emotional support Instruct client and family about disease process Instruct client and family about resources in the community	Most commonly arises in central airways Patient should be advised to quit smoking
Adenocarcinoma		
Weakness Anorexia Weight loss Shoulder pain Fever	Provide relief of dyspnea Provide pain management Instruct client in coughing techniques Provide emotional support for client and family Provide education about chemotherapeutic agents to client and family Provide nutritional support	Arises in peripheral lung tissue

Assessment Data	Nursing Interventions	Special Considerations
Large Cell		
Fever	Provide emotional support	
Weakness	Assist with pain management	
Anorexia		
Shoulder pain	Teach disease course	
Weight loss	Encourage adequate nutrition	
	Teach side effects of chemotherapeutic agents	
Small Cell		
Cough	Provide emotional support	May require intubation and mechanical ventilation
Dyspnea	Teach coughing techniques	
Hoarseness	Provide pain management	
Hemoptysis	Teach client about radiation therapy as indicated	
Chest pain	Provide pain management as indicated	
	Provide supplemental oxygen as indicated	
	Administer bronchodilator therapy as indicated	

Neuromuscular Alterations
Poliomyelitis

Acute poliomyelitis is a contagious disease that ranges from presentation of infection to paralytic illness and death. Three viral strains attack the motor cells of the anterior horn. Although vaccines have nearly eliminated the disease, it continues to occur in lower socioeconomic areas. Presentation may include flaccid/paralysis, diminished deep tendon reflexes, muscular wasting, and respiratory paralysis.

Assessment Data	Nursing Interventions	Special Considerations
Prodromal Stage		
Malaise	Assess vital signs	Incubation is 3 weeks
Low-grade fever	Monitor for signs of respiratory failure and increasing muscle weakness	
Coryza		Nursing goals are aimed at prevention of complications and deformities
GI disturbances		
CNS fluid:	Monitor for difficulty with swallowing, possible aspiration	
Increased WBC		
Increased protein		
Paralytic Stage		
Severe general symptoms		
Neck stiffness		
Pain		
Urine retention		
Fever of 39.5-40.5° C		
Collapse		
Coma		

Guillain-Barré Syndrome

Guillain-Barré syndrome (Landry-Guillain-Barré syndrome, Guillain-Barré-Strohl syndrome, acute polyneuritis, acute inflammatory polyradiculoneuropathy, or French polio) is a post infectious process thought to be a hypersensitivity or autoimmune response (Davis, 1979). Clients experience the syndrome 1 to 2 weeks following an upper respiratory infection or vaccination. The disease is characterized by a progressive muscular paralysis that begins in the periphery and moves centrally over a period of hours to days.

The paralysis may stop at any point or ascend through the cervical level. Prognosis is usually good; however, some clients may require intubation and mechanical ventilation in the face of respiratory failure secondary to muscular paralysis.

Assessment Data	Nursing Interventions	Special Considerations
Progressive weakness	Assess vital signs	Be alert for respiratory muscle fatigue
Motor disturbances	Assess respiratory pattern	
Parathesias	Maintain patent airway	Prepare for possible intubation and mechanical ventilation
Facial diplegia		
Dysphagia	Assess for increasing paralysis	
Loss of deep reflexes	Prevent complications secondary to muscle paralysis	Ensure that clients requiring mechanical ventilation are connected to their ventilators at all times
Muscular paralysis		
Nerve sensitivity to pressure	Provide comfort measures, e.g., frequent positioning and linen changes	
Profuse sweating		If ventilator disconnects, these clients lack ability to initiate respiration
Cerebrospinal fluid (CSF): Albuminocytologic dissociation	Provide constant observation for clients on mechanical ventilation	
		Has a long rehabilitation phase

Assessment Data	Nursing Interventions	Special Considerations
	Establish a method of communication, e.g., letterboard, wordboard, flashcards	

Amyotropic Lateral Sclerosis

Amyotropic lateral sclerosis (ALS) is characterized by a progressive muscular weakness that may involve the respiratory muscles. Early signs include weakness and muscle spasticity. The degenerative disease destroys the pyramidal tracts of the spinal cord and the motor cells.

Assessment Data	Nursing Interventions	Special Considerations
Fatigue	Assess vital signs	May require intubation and mechanical ventilation secondary to respiratory failure
Dsyphagia	Assess respiratory pattern	
Muscular weakness		
Muscular atrophy	Monitor for respiratory muscle fatigue and respiratory failure	
Spasticity of hands and arms		
	Observe for aspiration	

Myasthenia Gravis

Muscular fatigue is the primary characteristic of myasthenia gravis. The disease course includes periods of remission, exacerbation, and recovery. The muscular weakness and fatigue are thought to be the result of impaired neuromuscular transmission at the myoneural junction (Davis, 1979). Administration of anticholinesterase drugs are useful in symptom relief.

Assessment Data	Nursing Interventions	Special Considerations
Extraocular muscle weakness	Assess vital signs	Excerbations may result in respiratory muscle fatigue requiring intubation and mechanical ventilation
Ptosis	Assess respiratory pattern	
Diplopia	Observe for exacerbation	
Blurred vision		
Swallowing difficulty	Promote periods of rest	
Facial muscle weakness	Monitor for respiratory muscle fatigue and possible respiratory failure.	
Difficulty with speech		
Respiratory muscle fatigue		

Muscular Dystrophy

Muscular dystrophy (Duchenne's disease) is a congenital disease characterized by muscular degeneration and wasting. Initial involvement includes the muscles of the pelvic girdle.

Assessment Data	Nursing Interventions	Special Considerations
Bulky calf and forearm muscles	Assess respiratory status	Respiratory infection is frequently the cause of death
Waddling gait	Observe for signs of aspiration	
Muscular weakness		
Muscular atrophy	Provide support for limbs and trunk	
Respiratory failure	Suction airway to clear secretions	
	Observe for signs of respiratory infection	

Sleep Apnea

Sleep apnea is defined as the cessation of respiration for at least 10 seconds during sleep. Sleep apnea can be obstructive, central, or mixed (Boysen and Block, 1989). Obstructive apnea occurs when there is an obstruction in the pharynx. Thoracicabdominal movement continues despite absence of airflow. "Central apnea is an absence of airflow with no attempt to breathe" (Boysen and Block, 1989). Mixed apnea is a combination of brief periods of central apnea and upper airway obstruction. Short periods of sleep apnea are normal findings in healthy adults. The diagnosis of sleep apnea is made when the client has more than 30 periods of apnea during a 7-hour sleep interval. Sleep apnea usually produces hundreds of periods of apnea during a single sleeping period.

Assessment Data	Nursing Interventions	Special Considerations
Physical examination may be unremarkable	Assess vital signs	May require placement of tracheostomy tube to maintain patent airway
Systemic hypertension	Assess respiratory pattern	
Peripheral edema	Observe and document behavior during sleep	Nasal and mask continuous positive airway pressure (CPAP) have been effective treatment during sleep
Loud second heart sound	Monitor oxygen saturation via pulse oximetry during sleep	
Cor pulmonale by ECG		
Pulmonary function test (PFT) changes related to obesity	Assist client with weight reduction program	
Obesity		
Short, thick neck		
Obstructed nares		
Deviated nasal septum		
Loud snoring		

Assessment Data	Nursing Interventions	Special Considerations
Daytime somno-lence		
Morning headaches		
Nocturnal enuresis		
Personality changes		
Hypertension		
Intellectual deterio-ration		

Occupational Lung Disease
Pneumoconiosis

Pneumoconiosis is used to describe a number of respiratory conditions that cause inflammation, scarring, development of nodular lesions, and possible progression to diffuse pulmonary fibrosis (Springhouse, 1989b). Occupations at greatest risk for the development of pneumoconiosis are miners, textile mill workers, farmers, foundry workers, and stone cutters (See Table 3-1).

Table 3-1 Pneumoconiosis

Disease	Causative Agent	Source
Anthracosilicosis Coal workers' pneumoconiosis Black lung	Coal	Coal mining
Asbestosis	Asbestos	Mining; manufacturing tile; and roofing, fireproofing materials
Bird fancier's disease	Birds	Bird handlers
Carbon pneumoconiosis	Carbon Graphite	Manufacturing with black carbon (pencils, paint, ink, carbon paper, printing)
Diatomite silicosis	Diatomite	Mining diatomite Manufacturing bricks, cement
Siderosis	Iron	Iron and steel worker
Stannosis	Tin	Tin ore refinery worker
Silicosis	Silica	Mining precious metal Stonecutting Glass manufacturing
Talc pneumoconiosis	Talc	Manufacturing cosmetics and talc powder

(Adapted from Respiratory care handbook, Springhouse Corporation, Springhouse PA, 1989).

Silicosis

Silicosis is a progressive disease of the lung caused by inhalation of crystalline silica dust. Many workers involved in the manufacturing of glass, china, stoneware, and earthenware, as well as people who work with stonecutting and masonry, are at risk for silicosis. The disease is manifested by nodular lesions and progressive diffuse pulmonary fibrosis.

Assessment Data	Nursing Interventions	Special Considerations
History of exposure	Assess baseline respiratory function and ability to perform activities of daily living	A pulmonary rehabilitation program may be helpful in learning how to perform activities of daily living
Dyspnea on exertion		
Dry cough		
Tachypnea		
Decreased lung sounds	Instruct client and family in signs and symptoms of infection (fever, change in sputum color, consistency, amount, chills)	
Pulmonary hypertension		
PaO_2 normal or decreased		
$PaCO_2$ normal or decreased initially, rising as restrictive disease worsens	Encourage oral fluid intake of 3 L/day	
	Institute CPT/PD as appropriate	
	Instruct family in CPT/PD as indicated	
	Provide supplemental oxygen as ordered	
	Instruct family and client in pulmonary hygiene measures	

Black Lung

Black lung (coal workers' pneumoconiosis) is common in coal miners because of inhalation of coal dust particles smaller than 5 μ in diameter. It is a progressive nodular disease that can result in massive fibrosis.

Assessment Data	Nursing Interventions	Special Considerations
Exertional dyspnea	Assess respiratory status	May develop pulmonary tuberculosis
Productive cough	Assess vital signs	
Recurrent bronchpulmonary infections	Monitor sputum production	May require intubation and mechanical ventilation as disease progresses
Barrel chest	Monitor ABGs as indicated	
Hyperresonant lungs to percussion	Provide CPT/PD as indicated	Recommend pulmonary rehabilitation program as appropriate to teach alterations in activities of daily living
Decreased lung sounds	Encourage fluid intake of at least 3 L/day	
Crackles		
Wheezes	Administer bronchodilators and steroids as indicated	
Rhonchi		
Pulmonary hypertension		
Right ventricular hypertrophy	Supplemental oxygen may be indicated	
Cor pulmonale		
Small opacities on chest x-ray film	Instruct client and family in disease progress	
Pao_2 normal to decreased		
$Paco_2$ normal to decreased	Instruct client and family in pulmonary hygiene measures and CPT/PD as indicated	
Decreased vital capacity		
Decreased $FEV_{1.0}$		

Asbestosis

Asbestosis, caused by exposure to asbestos, is characterized by diffuse interstitial pulmonary fibrosis, pleural plaques, and cancer of the pleura. Smokers with asbestosis have an increased risk of lung cancer.

Assessment Data	Nursing Interventions	Special Considerations
History of exposure	Assess vital signs	May require mechanical ventilation as disease progresses
Crackles in the bases	Assess respiratory status	
Irregular, linear diffuse infiltrates on chest x-ray film	Provide supplemental oxygen as needed	
Chest x-ray examination: Pleural thickening Enlarged heart Obliteration of costal angles	Initiate CPT/PD as indicated	
	Monitor for upper respiratory infection (URI)	
Decreased $FEV_{1.0}$, FVC, TLC	Instruct client and family in pulmonary hygiene measures	
Decreased Pao_2		
Decreased $Paco_2$		

Emergent Injuries
Smoke Inhalation

"Pulmonary insufficiency resulting from heat and smoke inhalation is the major cause of mortality in the fire victim" (Demling, 1989). Injury to the lung is the result of chemicals and byproducts of the combustible materials contained in the smoke. Carbon monoxide exists in abundant proportions in smoke. The carbon monoxide binds with hemoglobin more readily than oxygen, resulting in hypoxemia and tissue hypoxia. Hydrogen cyanide, a byproduct of polyurethane production, acts in the same way.

Thermal injuries in the upper airway should be suspected in the client with facial burns. Thermal injury to the upper airway results in edema, erythema, and ulceration.

Chemical injuries are the result of toxic gases within the smoke. Gases interact with the mucosa to produce acid and alkaline changes, which cause irritation, edema, bronchospasm, and ulceration of the mucosal lining of the tracheobronchial tree.

Assessment Data	Nursing Interventions	Special Considerations
Carbon Monoxide		
History of carbon monoxide exposure	Maintain a patent airway	May require emergent intubation and mechanical ventilation
Headache	Assess vital signs, noting respiratory pattern, rate, and use of accessory muscles of respiration	
Dizziness		
Confusion		
Nausea		
Elevated carbohemoglobin levels	Provide supplemental oxygen as indicated	
Thermal Injury		
Facial burns	Maintain patent airway	May require emergent intubation or tracheostomy
Singed nasal hair	Assess vital signs	
Hoarseness	Monitor respiratory pattern	
Airway obstruction	Provide supplemental oxygen as indicated	
Chemical Injury		
Bronchospasm	Maintain patent airway	May require intubation and mechanical ventilation
Increased airway pressure	Assess vital signs	
Decreased Pa_{O_2}	Assess respiratory pattern	
	Provide supplemental oxygen as indicated	

Toxic Gas Inhalation (Tables 3-2 and 3-3)

Toxic gas inhalation can be caused by inhalation of smoke during a fire or inhalation of a direct chemical, such as those released in industrial accidents. Damage to the respiratory tract ranges from irritation to edema and inflammation.

Table 3-2   Toxic gas inhalation from combustion

Source	Gas	Effect
Wood, cotton, paper	Aldehydes	Lung and mucosal damage
Nylon	Ammonia	Mucosal irritation
Petroleum products	Benzene	Mucosal irritation
Polyurethane	Hydrogen cyanide	Respiratory failure
Polyvinylchloride	Hydrogen chloride	Mucosal irritation
Wallpaper, wood	Nitrogen dioxide	Pulmonary edema Bronchial irritation
Organic material	Carbon monoxide	Hypoxia
	Carbon dioxide	Stupor

Table 3-3   Noxious gases

Gas	Where Found	Effect
Chlorine	Chemical, plastics Swimming pools	Choking Coughing Pulmonary edema Exudative inflammatory bronchitis Oropharyngeal edema
Ammonia	Household cleaning agents Production of plastics, fertilizers, explosives	Chemical bronchitis Upper airway obstruction Pulmonary edema
Sulfur dioxide	Smelting byproduct Paper manufacturing	Nose and throat irritation Cough
Nitrogen oxides	Welding Grain silos	Few irritating effects Long-term parenchymal disease

Assessment Data	Nursing Interventions	Special Considerations
Phase I		
Sneezing	Remove client from source of exposure	
Coughing		
Choking		
Phase II (from 1-24 hours)		
Oropharyngeal edema	Maintain airway patency	May require intubation or tracheostomy
Upper airway obstruction	Administer humidified oxygen as indicated	
Airway plugging		

Assessment Data	Nursing Interventions	Special Considerations
Increased bronchial secretions	Administer bronchodilators as appropriate	
Bronchospasm	Monitor for hypoxemia by ABGs	

Phase III
(occurs after resolution of acute respiratory failure)

Coughing	Maintain airway patency	
Mild bronchospasm	Monitor respiratory pattern, rate	

Phase IV
(after 2-5 weeks)

Progressive shortness of breath	Assess vital signs	May develop bronchiolitis fibrosa obliterans
Fever	Maintain patent airway	
Nodular infiltrates on chest x-ray examination	Provide humidified oxygen as appropriate	
Pink, frothy sputum	Monitor respiratory pattern, rate	
Tachycardia	Provide care as outlined in Acute respiratory failure (ARF)	
Tachypnea		

Near Drowning

Many factors determine the course of the near-drowning victim's recovery: prior health; circumstances of the event; amount of water aspirated; and phase of respiratory cycle, e.g., inhalation or exhalation (Modell and Boysen, 1989). Near drowning in cold water (below 20° C) elicits the mammalian diving reflex resulting in total body hypothermia. This state decreases oxygen consumption and has resulted in successful resuscitation of victims.

Aspiration of salt water produces fluid-filled alveoli and large intrapulmonary shunts due to the hyperosmolality of the fluid ingested. Fresh water aspiration floods the alveoli with hypoosmolar fluid resulting in unstable alveoli, which results in hypoxia and intrapulmonary shunting. Both salt and fresh water cause pulmonary edema.

Assessment Data	Nursing Interventions	Special Considerations
History of submersion	Assess vital signs	Prepare for possible intubation and mechanical ventilation
Dyspnea	Provide airway maintenance	
Apnea	Monitor oxygenation	
Pink, frothy sputum		Cardiopulmonary arrest is not uncommon
Decreased Pao_2	Administer supplemental oxygen as indicated	
Crackles		Prepare for possible CVP or PA catheter insertion
Wheezes	Assess respiratory pattern and rate	
Tachycardia		
Brachycardia	Monitor cardiac rhythm	
Asystole		
Initial rise in central venous pressure (CVP) and rapid return to normal	Monitor hemodynamics, if appropriate	

Thoracic Trauma

Thoracic injuries include a multitude of insults that occur directly to the thorax, and indirectly, through the thorax to the lung itself. Thoracic injuries can occur from falls, automobile accidents, and many other accidents that result in individual injury.

Pulmonary Contusion

Pulmonary contusions are the result of high-velocity impact with a dull object such as the edge of a table or the steering wheel of a car.

Assessment Data	Nursing Interventions	Special Considerations
Bruising of chest wall	Assess vital signs	May require chest tube if large amount of bleeding occurs.
Hemoptysis	Assess respiratory function	
History of high impact event	Monitor sputum for blood	Clients are at increased risk for developing ARDS
Decreased blood pressure	Teach client splinting techniques for coughing and deep breathing	
Tachycardia		
Tachypnea		
Hypotension		

Rib Fractures

Fractures of the ribs can be classified as simple (involving breakage of a single rib) or complex (involving multiple ribs and surrounding tissue).

Assessment Data	Nursing Interventions	Special Considerations
Bruising of thorax	Assess vital signs	May develop atelectasis secondary to decreased lung expansion
Pain on inspiration	Assess respiratory pattern for intracostal retraction	
Crackles		
Hemoptysis	Observe for hemoptysis	
Pulmonary contusion	Encourage deep breathing and coughing	
Tachycardia		
Tachypnea		
Hypotension		

Flail Chest

A flail chest is the breaking of two or more adjacent ribs in three or more places resulting in a free-floating section of thorax. The free-floating thoracic section moves paradoxically with inspiration and expiration. The client has increased work of breathing and hypoxia that result from the underlying pulmonary contusion.

Assessment Data	Nursing Interventions	Special Considerations
Flailing chest	Stabilize chest wall with sandbag or direct pressure	May require intubation and mechanical ventilation
Tachypnea		
Tachycardia	Assess vital signs	
Falling Pao$_2$	Monitor respiratory pattern	
Bruising over thorax		
Tenderness of thorax on palpation	Observe for intracostal retraction	
Hemoptysis		
Hypotension		

Pneumothorax

A pneumothorax occurs as the result of an accumulation of air or fluid within the thorax. Pneumothorax can result from a tear in the pleura, an open wound of the thorax, or bleeding into the pleural cavity from thoracic trauma. A tension pneumothorax is life-threatening and requires emergent intervention. Other pneumothoraxes may not produce symptoms unless they occupy 40% of the thorax or are involved with cardiopulmonary disease.

Tension Pneumothorax

A tension pneumothorax is life-threatening and requires immediate intervention. The buildup of air in the thorax occurs as air enters the pleural space through a tear in the pleural cavity, increasing tension in the chest; shifting the mediastinum to the unaffected side. If the tension is not relieved, cardiac arrest can result.

Assessment Data	Nursing Interventions	Special Considerations
Tension Pneumothorax		
Severe dyspnea	Support respiration	Prepare for immediate chest decompression
Increased airway pressure	If on mechanical ventilation disconnect; use self-inflating bag to support respirations	
Severe chest pain		Airway pressures will be reduced by disconnecting the client from the mechanical ventilator
Tachycardia		
Tachypnea		
Hypotension	Observe for arrhythmias	
Tracheal deviation	Monitor heart rate	May develop electromechanical dissociation
Decreased/absent lung sounds		
Cyanosis		
Open Pneumothorax		
Severe dyspnea	Maintain adequate airway	Prepare for chest decompression
Chest pain	Assess vital signs	
Crepitus	Monitor respiratory pattern	
Decreased or absent lung sounds		
Hyperresonance		
Closed Pneumothorax		
Increasing dyspnea	Assess vital signs	May require insertion of chest tube
Pleuritic-type chest pain	Monitor respiratory pattern	
Decreased lung expansion	Maintain positioning to maximize chest expansion	
Decreased lung sounds	Elevate head of bed	
Resonance or hyperresonance	Assess for subcutaneous emphysema	

Hemothorax

Hemothorax is defined as blood accumulation within the pleural space. The severity of the hemothorax is depends on the volume of blood loss and the rate of intrathoracic bleeding (Moser and Spragg 1982).

Assessment Data	Nursing Interventions	Special Considerations
History of thoracic trauma or invasive procedure	Monitor vital signs Assess respiratory status	May require intubation and mechanical ventilation
Increasing dyspnea	Administer fluid and blood replacement as ordered	Prepare for thoracentesis
Chest pain		
Tachycardia		
Tachypnea	Monitor hemodynamics	
Hypotension	Maintain chest tubes	
Dullness to percussion		

Postoperative Complications
Atelectasis

Atelectasis is an area of lung that has collapsed from excessive fluid in the alveloi, excessive secretions, proximal plugging, or alveolar hypoventilation. Most often it occurs postoperatively in clients who are overweight or immobile or do not breathe deeply because of chest discomfort.

Assessment Data	Nursing Interventions	Special Considerations
Coughing	Assess vital signs	In severe lobar collapse, tracheal deviation to the affected side may develop
Decreased breath sounds	Monitor respiratory pattern	
Dyspnea	Provide CPT/PD to affected area	
Wheezing		
Tachypnea	Encourage increased fluids	

Assessment Data	Nursing Interventions	Special Considerations
	Administer incentive spirometry three to four times per day	
	Increase mobility	
	Instruct in coughing techniques	
	Position on side with ateletic area up	

Pulmonary Emboli

Pulmonary emboli, obstruction of the pulmonary artery bed, is most often caused by deep vein thrombosis. Clients at risk for pulmonary emboli include those on prolonged bed rest, those who are obese or over 40 years old, and those who have a history of vascular disease or a chronic medical problem such as COPD, heart disease, or diabetes mellitus.

Assessment Data	Nursing Interventions	Special Considerations
Coughing	Assess vital signs	Pneumatic compression devices may be indicated to reduce the risk of deep vein thrombosis in those clients at increased risk for development of pulmonary emboli
Dyspnea	Monitor respiratory pattern	
Pleural friction rub		
Hypotension	Provide supplemental oxygen as indicated	
Hypoxia		
Blood-tinged sputum	Monitor ABGs or pulse oximetry as needed	
Tachycardia		
Anginal or pleuritic chest pain	Provide emotional support	
Decreased Pa_{CO_2}	Elevate head of bed 30-45 degrees	
S_3 gallop		

Assessment Data	Nursing Interventions	Special Considerations
Crackles	Provide thigh-high antiembolic stockings as ordered	
ECG changes		
Right bundle branch block		
Tall-peaked P waves	Administer thrombolytic agents as indicated	
Right axis deviation	Monitor for signs of bleeding and bruising	

Fat Emboli

Fat emboli produce a syndrome similar to ARDS. Fat globules originating from traumatic tissue embolize into the pulmonary capillaries, where the enzymatic breakdown releases fatty acid that irritates the lung. Most commonly, fat emboli are seen in clients with long bone fractures. (Burton and Hodgkin, 1984). See the discussion of ARDS for assessment findings, nursing interventions and special considerations.

Thoracic Surgery

Clients undergo a number of surgical procedures for treatment of lung disease. The following summarizes the most common procedures, their purpose, and postoperative nursing considerations.

Procedure	Purpose	Postoperative Nursing Considerations
Thoracotomy Opening of the thorax	Exploration	Chest tubes
	Diagnosis	Coughing/deep breathing
	Lung cancer	
Pneumonectomy Removal of an entire lung	Trauma	No chest tubes
	Removal of tumors	Coughing/deep breathing
Lobectomy Removal of a lobe of the lung	Bronchiectasis	One or two chest tubes
	Emphysematous blebs	

Procedure	Purpose	Postoperative Nursing Considerations
Wedge resection: Removal of a well-defined diseased area	Abscesses	Coughing/deep breathing
	Localized tumors	Chest tubes
	Local inflammatory disease	Chest tubes
Segmental resection: Removal of one or more lobar segments	Bronchiectasis	Coughing/deep breathing
	Abscesses	Chest tubes
	Tumor	Coughing/deep breathing
Decortication: Stripping a thick, fibrous membrane from the visceral pleura	Chronic emphysema	
	Failure of chest to reexpand after resection	No chest tubes
		Coughing/deep breathing
Thoracoplasty: Removal of ribs to decrease size of thoracic cavity		

Lung Transplantation

Lung transplantation was successfully performed in 1983 by Dr. Joel Cooper in Toronto, Canada. Although it is a relatively new procedure, it is more frequently being attempted at major medical centers throughout the United States and in Europe. Today, single and double lung transplants occur independent of the heart.

Interstitial pulmonary fibrosis, emphysema caused by alpha$_1$-antitrypsin deficiency, cystic fibrosis, and primary pulmonary hypertension are the diseases accepted for transplantation. Candidates for lung transplantation must undergo cardiopulmonary stress testing, right ventriculograms, cardiac catheterization, full pulmonary function testing, chest radiography, and a complete battery of blood tests.

Acceptance into a program requires that candidates complete an extensive pulmonary rehabilitation program. The candidates are given an exercise prescription and monitored throughout their workout sessions. Exercises include stretching and strengthening exercises, chest mobility exercises, biking, walking on a treadmill, and arm ergometry. The candidates are monitored with pulse oximetry to assess heart rate and oxygen saturation. Oxygen therapy is adjusted to maintain saturations of arterial oxygen of more than 85%. Physical therapy is evaluated to assist with the mobilization and joint problems as necessary.

The candidate also attends a series of classes about lung transplantation, complications, risk factors, medications, expected course of treatment, pulmonary hygiene, and candidate commitment. A strenuous pulmonary hygiene program is initiated, including hydration, chest physiotherapy, postural drainage, vibration, rib shaking, bronchodilitation, and aerosol therapy.

Single lung transplantation is performed when the remaining lung is stiff and noncompliant. Since air travels into the lung with the least resistance, the transplanted lung receives the ventilation. Double lung transplantation is used in lung diseases in which the remaining lung would be floppy and offer no resistance. Experimentally, single lung transplantations are being performed with success in candidates with emphysema who would usually have received a double lung transplant.

The postoperative course is comprised of rehabilitation and evaluation for rejection. If candidates do well, they usually are extubated and taken out of the intensive care unit within 4 to 5 days. Immediately the exercise and rehabilitation phase begins. The success of the preoperative program has a direct effect on the postoperative course. Severely compromised candidates have returned to normal functional ability in activities of daily living. Some complications of lung transplantation are dehiscence of the airway, or anastomosis; rejection of the new organ; bronchieolitis obliterans; and opportunistic infections caused by immunosuppressive drug therapy.

References

Boyson PG and Block AJ: Cardiopulmonary consequences of sleep and breathing disorders. In Shoemaker WC et al: Textbook of critical care, Philadelphia, 1989, WB Saunders Co.

Burton GG and Hodgkin JE: Respiratory care, a guide to clinical practice, ed 2, Philadelphia, 1984, JB Lippincott Co.

Davis JE and Mason CB: Neurological critical care, Atlanta, 1979, Van Nostrand Reinhold Company.

Demling RH: Management of the burn patient. In Shoemaker WC, et al: Textbook of critical care, Philadelphia, 1989, WB Saunders Co.

Groenwald SL, ed: Cancer nursing, principles and practice, Boston, 1987, Jones and Bartlett Publishers Inc.

Modell JH and Boysen PG: Drowning and near-drowning. In Shoemaker WC et al: Textbook of critical care, Philadelphia, 1989, WB Saunders Co.

Moser KM and Spragg RG: Respiratory emergencies, ed 2, St. Louis, 1982, The CV Mosby Co.

Petty TL: Acute respiratory failure in chronic obstructive pulmonary disease. In Shoemaker WC, et al: Textbook of critical care, Philadelphia, 1989, WB Saunders Co.

Springhouse Nursing 85 Books: Clinical pocket manual respiratory care, Springhouse Corporation, 1989 Springhouse, Pa.

Springhouse Nursing 85 Books: Respiratory care handbook, Springhouse Corporation, 1989, Springhouse, Pa.

Bibliography

Boyda E: Respiratory problems, Oradell. NF, 1985, Medical Economics Books.

Chusid JG: Correlative neuroanatomy and functional neurology, Los Altos, Calif, 1982, Lange Medical Books.

Farer LS: Tuberculosis: what the physician should know, American Lung Association and its medical section American Thoracic Society, 1986.

Heimbecker RO et al: Heart and heart-lung transplantation, Heart Lung 13(1), 1984.

Montefusco CM and Veith FJ: Lung transplantation, Surg Clin North Am 66(3):503-15,1986.

Murray JF and Nadel, JA: Textbook of respiratory medicine, Vols I & II, Philadelphia, 1988, WB Saunders Co.

Perry AG and Potter PA, eds: Shock comprehensive nursing management, St.Louis, 1983, The C.V. Mosby Co.

Seaton A et al: Respiratory diseases, ed 4, Blackwell Scientific Publications Inc. 1989.

Shoemaker WC et al: Textbook of critical care, Philadelphia, 1989, WB Saunders Co.

Veith FJ: Lung transplantation in perspective, New Engl J Med 314(18):1186-1187, 1986 (editorial).

Wyngaarden JB and Smith LH: Cecil textbook of medicine, vol 1, ed 16, Philadelphia, 1982, WB Saunders Co.

Airway Management

4

Artificial Airways

Maintaining airway patency is critical in managing clients with respiratory alterations. Patency can be accomplished through the use of oral airways, endotracheal and tracheostomy tubes, and procedures such as suctioning and chest physiotherapy, which help clear airway secretions.

Oropharyngeal Airways (see Fig. 4-1)

Proper oropharyngeal airway size is determined by measuring the distance from the corner of the client's mouth to the angle of the jaw below the ear. This length should be equal to the distance from the flange of the airway to the tip. The airway may be easily dislodged or stimulate gagging if it is too large.

Insertion Techniques	Nursing Considerations
Insert the oral airway upside down in the mouth and rotate into position (Fig. 4-2).	Pushing the oral airway into the mouth will displace the tongue into the posterior pharynx, occluding the airway
Use a tongue depressor to hold the tongue in place. Insert the airway into the mouth	

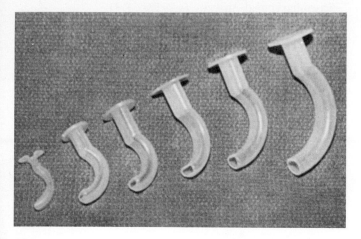

Figure 4-1
Oropharyngeal airways.
(From Abels LF: Mosby's manual of critical care, St Louis, 1979, The CV Mosby Co).

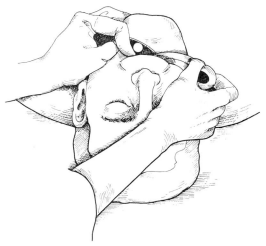

Figure 4-2
Rotating the airway into place.
(From Abels LF: Mosby's manual of critical care, St Louis, 1979, The CV Mosby Co).

Nasopharyngeal Airways (see Fig. 4-3)

When selecting an airway it is important to choose one that is the appropriate size for the client. The usual size for an adult is a 7 mm or 8 mm airway.

Insertion Techniques	Nursing Considerations
Lubricate airway with water-soluble lubricant.	Airway should be rotated from nare to nare every 8 hours to prevent necrosis
Insert into patent nares.	
Tip should lie in posterior pharynx (Fig. 4-4)	Assess for patency and pressure sores every 4 hours
	If other nare is occluded with secretions or secondary to edema, assess airway patency hourly

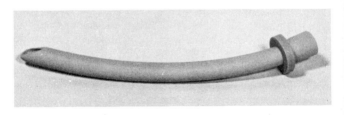

Figure 4-3
Nasopharyngeal airway.
(From Sheehy S: Emergency nursing, St Louis, 1985, The CV Mosby Co).

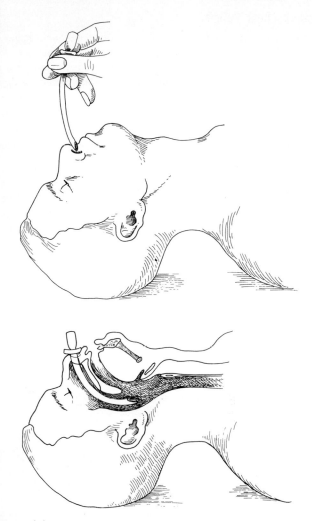

Figure 4-4

Insertion of the nasopharyngeal airway.
(From Abels LF: Mosby's manual of critical care, St Louis, 1979, The CV Mosby Co).

Endotracheal Tubes

Endotracheal tubes (ETT) are indicated for clients who cannot protect their airway, to assist in removal of pulmonary secretions, and to allow respiratory management with positive pressure ventilation (Fig. 4-5). Endotracheal tubes are placed nasally or orally (see Emergency management: assisting with ETT insertion) (Fig. 4-6). The average adult size ETT is 7.5 to 9.0 mm. (See Table 4-1.) Along the length of the ETT, centimeter markings indicate the level of tube insertion. The average adult tube is placed at 24 to 26 cm at the lips.

Endotracheal tubes should be repositioned every 24 hours, alternating sides of the mouth. Cloth tape can be used to secure the ETT and is changed daily or as needed. It is positioned across the cheeks and upper lip; taping across the lower jaw and chin increases the chance of self-extubation caused by chewing on the tube and jaw movement (Fig. 4-7). Commercially prepared endotracheal tube holders are also available.

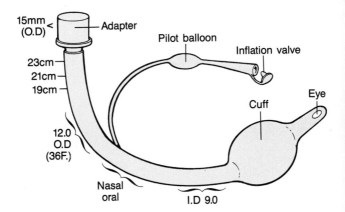

Figure 4-5
Endotracheal tube.

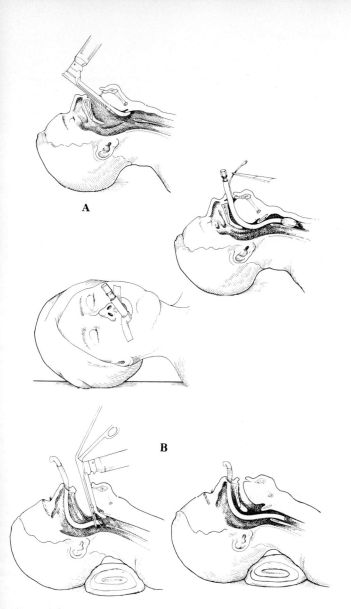

Figure 4-6
Endotracheal tube placement **A,** Oral tracheal tube; **B,** Nasal tracheal tube.

(From Abels LF: Mosby's manual of critical care, St Louis, 1979, The CV Mosby Co).

Table 4-1 Endotracheal tube sizes

Client Age	Recommended ETT Size (ID)	Position Level
12 years	6.5 mm	22 cm
16 years	7.0 mm	23 cm
Adult male	8.0-9.0 mm	24-25 cm
Adult female	7.5-8.5 mm	25-26 cm

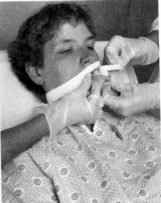

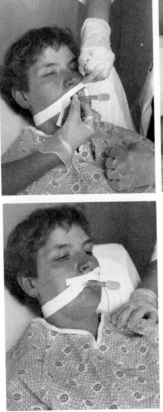

Figure 4-7
Taping the oral endotracheal tube.
(From Perry A and Potter P: Clinical nursing skills and techniques, ed 2, St Louis, 1990, The CV Mosby Co).

Changing ETT tape requires two clinicians, one to hold the tube in place, noting the centimeter level, and the other to secure the tube in position with the tape. The following procedure is used:

1. Tear a piece of tape approximately 20 inches long.
2. Place a 6-inch piece of tape in the center of a 20-inch piece, sticky sides together.
3. Slide tape behind client's head, centering nonsticky area behind head from ear to ear.
4. Prepare cheeks by washing. Shave client if necessary. Dry thoroughly.
5. Apply tincture of benzoin to cheeks and under nose.
6. Bring length of tape across face at cheek level.
7. Split tape in half. Bring lower half across upper lip.
8. Wrap other half two or three times around ETT and then back onto client's cheek.
9. Do not pull tape so taut as to cause tension on the client's face. Repeat on opposite side.

Meticulous oral care is required every 2 to 4 hours for clients with an ETT in place. Observe the oral mucosa for signs of ulcerations and areas of necrosis, especially on the posterior tongue and at the corners of the mouth.

Endobronchial Tubes

Endobronchial tubes (Figs. 4-8 to 4-10) are special tubes used to selectively intubate the right and left mainstem bronchus for independent lung ventilation. These tubes allow separate ventilation of each lung and protection of one lung from aspirate from the other, as in massive hemoptysis.

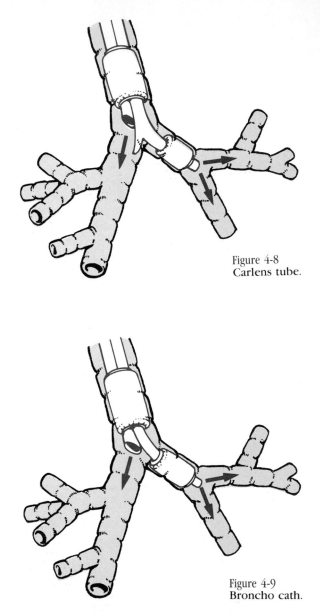

Figure 4-8
Carlens tube.

Figure 4-9
Broncho cath.

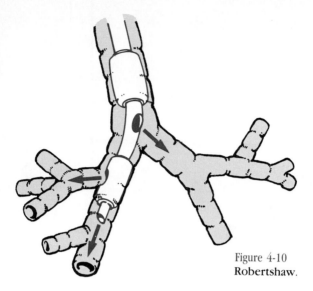

Figure 4-10
Robertshaw.

Tracheostomy Tubes

Tracheostomy tubes are used for long-term airway management or prolonged mechanical ventilation. Many types of tracheostomy tubes are available from various manufacturers (see Table 4-2). Size is determined by inner diameter, not exterior diameter. Table 4-3 lists various tracheostomy tubes by size, listing both internal and external diameters for comparison and conversion from one manufacturer to another.

Tracheostomy care should always be sterile for the first 72 hours following the procedure and for those clients who are infected or immunosuppressed. Clean tracheostomy care using good medical asepsis will provide the client with adequate infection control (Table 4-4). Clinicians should follow institutional policy. Clients with tracheostomies should be taught self-care as soon as medically feasible.

Table 4-2 Tracheostomy tube types

Type of Tube	Indications	Nursing Considerations
Cuffed, no inner cannula (Fig. 4-11)	Airway management Positive pressure ventilation Small to moderate amount of secretions	Tracheostomy care every 4 to 6 hours. Single cannula could become clogged. This would be life-threatening and require changing the tube immediately.

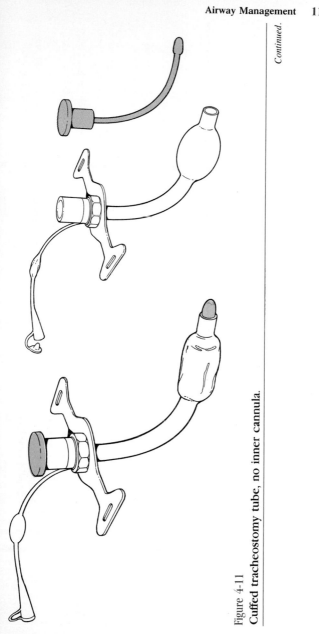

Continued.

Figure 4-11
Cuffed tracheostomy tube, no inner cannula.

Table 4-2 Tracheostomy tube types—cont'd

Type of Tube	Indications	Nursing Considerations
Cuffed, permanent/ disposable inner cannula (Fig. 4-12)	Airway management Positive pressure ventilation Large amount of secretions	Tracheostomy care every 4 to 6 hours. Change inner cannula with tracheostomy care and as needed. While permanent inner cannula is being cleaned, there is no way to connect client to ventilator, unless a second inner cannula is obtained. Disposable inner cannulas reduce nursing time.
Metal (Fig. 4-13)	Long-term airway maintenance	Usually cuffless. Needs to be removed completely at least once a week and cleaned Inner cannula care is done every 6 to 8 hours Hydrogen peroxide should not be used on silver-plated or stainless steel, since it oxidizes the metal, causing pitting and flaking of the tube.

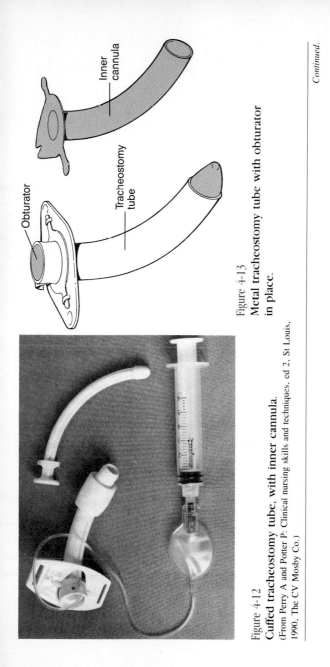

Figure 4-12
Cuffed tracheostomy tube, with inner cannula.
(From Perry A and Potter P: Clinical nursing skills and techniques, ed 2, St Louis, 1990, The CV Mosby Co.)

Figure 4-13
Metal tracheostomy tube with obturator in place.

Continued.

Table 4-2 Tracheostomy tube types—cont'd

Type of Tube	Indications	Nursing Considerations
Cuffless/disposable	Long-term airway maintenance For clients who are allergic or do not tolerate metal tube.	Should be changed every 4 weeks. Inner cannula care should be performed every 6 to 8 hours.
Fenestrated cuffed/cuffless (Fig. 4-14)	Long-term airway maintenance Intermittent access to airway; can be plugged and client can talk	If the tracheostomy tube is plugged, the cuff *must* be deflated for adequate ventilation. Can also be used in the client who is hard to wean.

Continued.

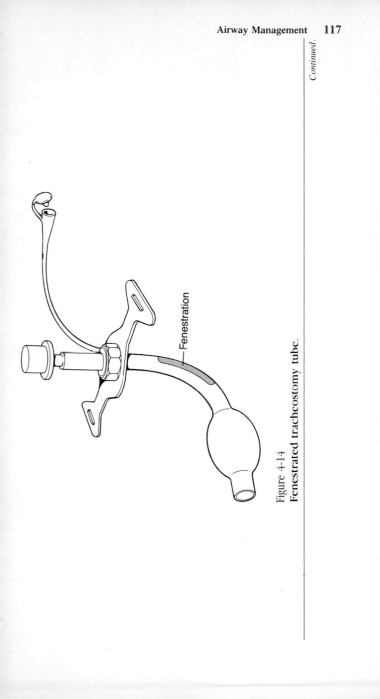

Figure 4-14
Fenestrated tracheostomy tube.

Table 4-2 Tracheostomy tube types—cont'd

Type of Tube	Indications	Nursing Considerations
Speaking tracheostomy tube	Allows client to use voice	Requires manual dexterity on the part of the client to operate air insufflation port. May increase client frustration and depression with regard to inability to communicate easily. Small cuffs are more difficult to seal.
Double-cuffed tube	Alternately inflated cuffs help reduce tracheal damage	
Fome cuff (Fig. 4-15)	Long-term care Difficult to seal tracheostomy Decreases tracheal necrosis	Cuff inflation port must be left open to assure cuff filling by negative pressure. Cuff must be aspirated every 8 hours to remove any fluid that may have been drawn into cuff. Tube should be changed every 4 weeks. Leaving tube in place longer may result in difficulty in deflating cuff for removal.

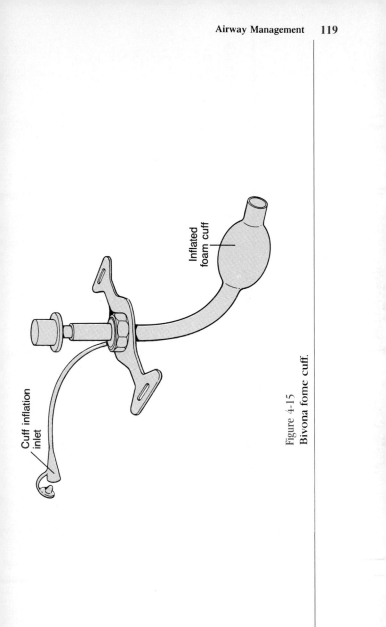

Cuff inflation
inlet

Inflated
foam cuff

Figure 4-15
Bivona fome cuff.

Table 4-3   Comparison of tracheostomy tube sizes by manufacturer

Size	Portex DIC ID/OD*	Portex ID/OD*	Shiley† ID/OD*	Jackson ID/OD*	KW Fome	French
4				5.5/8.0		24
5			5.0/8.5	6.0-6.5/9	6.0/8.7	27
6	6.0/8.5	6.0/8.1		7.0/10	7/10	30
7	7.0/9.9	7.0/9.7	7.0/10.0	7.5-8.0/11	8/11	33
8	8.0/11.3	8.0/11.0	8.5/12.0	8.5/12	9.0/12.3	36
9	9.0/12.6	9.0/12.1		9.0-9.5/13		39
10	10.0/14.0	10.0/13.5	9.0/13.0	10.0/14		42

*Millimeters
†Includes disposable inner cannulas

Table 4-4 Tracheostomy care

Frequency	Supplies	Procedure
Single Cannula		
6-8 hr	Gloves Hydrogen peroxide Sterile saline 4 × 4 tracheal dressing Tracheostomy ties	Clean area around stoma Replace trachea flat and tracheostomy ties
Double Cannula		
4-6 hr	Gloves Hydrogen peroxide Sterile saline Tracheostomy brush or disposable inner cannula Tracheostomy ties	Remove and clean inner cannula. (If disposable inner cannula is used, simply replace with new.) Clean area around stoma. Replace trachea flat and tracheostomy ties.
Metal		
4-6 hr	Gloves Sterile saline Instrument cleanser (e.g., Manucleanser, Vestal V5) Tracheostomy brush Tracheostomy ties	Remove and clean inner cannula. Clean area around stoma. Replace inner cannula. Replace trachea flat and tracheostomy ties.

Changing tracheostomy ties

1. Measure the distance from the tracheostomy tube from behind the neck and then back to the tracheostomy tube. Cut a tracheostomy tie two times this length.
2. Untie one side of the soiled tracheostomy tie.
3. Make sure to hold the tracheostomy tube in place while removing the old ties and replacing them with the new ties.
4. Thread the end of the new tracheostomy tie through the slot on the flange of the tracheostomy tube.
5. Pull through until the ends of the tie are even.
6. Straighten the ties and adjust behind the client's neck.
7. Remove the soiled tracheostomy tie from the opposite side of the tracheostomy tube.
8. Thread the end of one side of the tracheostomy tie through the slot on the flange of the tracheostomy tube.
9. Tie the two ends together at the side of the neck with a square knot.
10. Be sure to allow one finger space between the neck and the secured tie.

Table 4-5 lists accessories available for use with tracheostomy tubes.

Table 4-5   Tracheostomy accessories

Accessories	Purpose	Nursing Considerations
Tracheostomy plug	Allows plugging of tracheostomy tube for client to speak	Be sure to have tracheostomy cuff deflated.
Kisner button	Allows client to speak while maintaining open stoma	Needs to be cleaned frequently to prevent valve sticking.
Tracheostomy button (Fig. 4-16)	Replaces tracheostomy Maintains open stoma	Can be unbuttoned to allow suctioning.

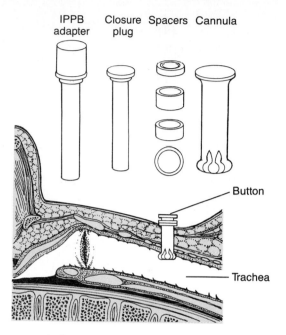

Figure 4-16
Tracheostomy button.

Managing a Cuffed Tube

The care of ETT and tracheostomy tubes with cuffs is the same. Current tube cuffs are usually high volume-low pressure cuffs that prevent tracheal wall damage by distributing the cuff pressure over a large surface area.

A cuff seal is maintained by inflating the cuff to a volume that allows the client to achieve the prescribed tidal volume when on a mechanical ventilator, when no leak of air is ausculated over the trachea, or until 18 mm of mercury is reached. Minimal cuff leak techniques are achieved by sealing the cuff and then aspirating 0.1 ml of air. This helps to reduce possible tracheal necrosis. Cuff leaks of less than 50 ml of tidal volume are generally acceptable as long as the client's physiologic parameters remain stable. Measuring cuff pressure can be accomplished with an aneroid cuff pressure manometer or a syringe, stopcock, and blood pressure manometer (Fig. 4-17).

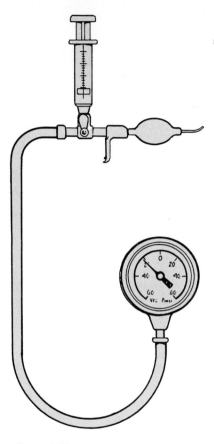

Figure 4-17
Measuring cuff pressure.

1. Assemble three-way stopcock, 12 ml syringe, and blood pressure manometer.
2. Place stopcock on end of blood pressure (BP) tubing.
3. Attach pilot balloon of cuffed tube to port directly opposite the port attached to the BP tubing.
4. Set syringe plunger at 5 ml.
5. Attach syringe to remaining side port of the stopcock.
6. Open stopcock between syringe and BP manometer.
7. Insert 1-2 ml of air into BP manometer.
8. Allow air to equilibrate with BP manometer at 0.
9. Open stopcock to pilot balloon and close to the syringe.
10. Observe pressure on BP manometer.
11. If pressure is greater than 18 mm Hg, open to syringe and withdraw .5 ml of air.
12. Remeasure cuff pressure.
13. If pressure is less than 18 mm Hg, only add air if cuff seal is inadequate.

The clinician caring for clients with ETT or tracheostomy tubes should assess the client frequently for complications. Table 4-6 lists the most frequent complications.

Table 4-6 Complications with ETT/tracheostomy tubes

Clinical Presentation	Problem	Nursing Considerations
Client complains of difficulty breathing. Difficulty in suctioning. Inability to advance suction catheter	Tube lumen obstructed or herniated cuff blocking distal end of tube	Use ambu bag and attempt suctioning. Instill NS to help loosen obstruction. Replace tube.
Sudden large airleak Low-pressure alarm of ventilator sounds Client's exhaled V_T decreases	Ruptured cuff	Replace tube immediately. Support respiration with ambu bag.
Unequal or unilateral chest wall expansions (ETT)	Dislodged tube	Determine level of ETT by checking cm marking. Reposition tube with physician's assistance.

Client is able to vocalize		
Decreased or absent breath sounds on the left side		Replace tube. Assess client's ability to ventilate adequately.
Tracheostomy tube is completely out of place and client is having difficulty breathing		Reposition tube if applicable.
High pressure alarm on ventilator sounds	Kinking of tube	Reposition tube. Replace tube if kink cannot be straightened.

Suctioning

Suctioning of the tracheobronchial tree is necessary for many clients with increased pulmonary secretions (see Table 4-7). The removal of airway secretions is a strict aseptic technique using double gloves. The suctioning procedure is performed based on assessment of the client's breath sounds. Suctioning should not exceed 10 to 15 seconds. Actual application of suction is only performed during withdrawal of the catheter and should not exceed 10 seconds (Holloway, 1988). Suction pressures greater than 80 to 120 mm Hg may be associated with damage to the tracheobronchial mucosa.

The most common complication of suctioning is hypoxemia. Clients who are receiving an FiO_2 of greater than 40% may benefit from hyperventilation, hyperinflation, and hyperoxygenation before suctioning.

Hyperventilation	Use ambu bag 4 to 6 times before suctioning
	Helps to open alveoli
	Usually delivers V_T 700-900 ml
Hyperinflation	Achieved by ventilating at 1½ times the tidal volume
	Can be accomplished by using the sigh volume on the volume ventilator
	Can be accomplished with the ambu bag when the tidal volume is small
Hyperoxygenation	Provide 1½ to 2 minutes of 100% oxygen before suctioning
	Reduces hypoxemia associated with suctioning

Other complications associated with suctioning include cardiac arrhythmias, increased shortness of breath, anxiety of the client, and bronchospasm or laryngospasm. Assess the client's breath sounds, vital signs, and other possible complications after suctioning is completed. Always take time to reassure the client and allow him or her to relax. At least 20 to 30 seconds should elapse between suction passes. If hyperoxygenation has been used, ensure that the prescribed oxygen concentration has been restored to the client.

The technique for suctioning is as follows (Perry, 1990):

1. Wash hands.
2. Turn suction on and regulate pressure.
3. Open suction kit.
4. Open suction catheter maintaining sterility.
5. Apply sterile glove to dominant hand and clean glove to nondominant hand.
6. Pick up suction catheter with sterile gloved hand.
7. Using clean gloved hand, pick up connecting tubing and assemble with suction catheter.
8. Expose artificial airway.
9. Preoxygenate and/or hyperinflate client with assistance from second clinician.
10. Gently insert catheter until resistance is met.
11. Withdraw catheter and rotate, intermittently applying suction.
12. Allow client 20 to 30 seconds to rest between suction passes.
13. If catheter is clogged, rinse with sterile water before repeating procedure.

Oral/pharyngeal suction

Oral/pharyngeal suction is used in clients who have difficulty in swallowing or who have excessive oral secretions. Suctioning prevents aspiration of secretions into the lower airway. A Yankauer or tonsillar tip suction device is used. The suction device is rigid plastic and should be made of clear material, which allows for visualization of the aspirated secretions.

The catheter is inserted gently into the mouth. Secretions are removed through many holes at the tip of the catheter. Suction pressure is constant, since there is no port for regulation of suction (Fig. 4-18).

Suction catheters

The size of the suction catheter used should be no greater than one half the size of the internal diameter of the endotracheal tube or the tracheostomy tube. (Zschoche, 1985). Table 4-8 lists recommended suction catheter sizes for ETT or tracheostomy tubes.

Table 4-7 Comparison of suctioning procedures

	Nasal/Oral Pharyngeal	Nasal/Oral Tracheal	Endotracheal/Tracheostomy
Technique	Sterile	Sterile	Sterile
Suction pressure	80-120 mm Hg	80-120 mm Hg	80-120 mm Hg
Insertion depth	6 cm in adults: distance from tip of nose to base above ear lobe	20-24 cm in adults	20-24 cm in adults
Suction time	10 seconds	10 seconds	10 seconds
Special considerations	Lubricate 6-8 cm of distal end of catheter with water-soluble lubricant Allow 1-2 minutes between suction passes if client is not receiving supplemental oxygen	Lubricate 6-8 cm of distal end of catheter with water-soluble lubricant Catheter size: 12-16 French in adult; advance catheter during inspiration	Water-soluble lubricant may be used Evaluate need to preoxygenate and hyperventilate before suctioning

As epiglottis is open and will facilitate passage into trachea

Use downward slant to avoid turbinates when nasal route is used.

Allow 1-2 minutes between suction passes if client is not receiving supplemental oxygen (Perry and Potter, 1990)

Instillation of 5-10 ml of sterile saline may help thin secretions in the artificial airway

Normal saline instillation has little effect on airway secretions in the tracheobronchial tree (Ackerman, 1985)

(Adapted from Perry A and Potter P: Clinical nursing skills and techniques, ed 2, St Louis, 1990, The CV Mosby Co)

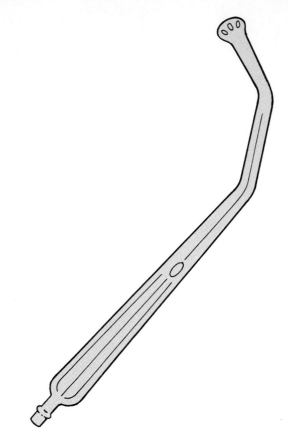

Figure 4-18
Yankauer suction.

Table 4-8   Suction catheter sizes for ETT/tracheostomy tubes

Tube Size	Suction Catheter Size
(ID mm)	(French)
6.0	10
6.5	10
7.0	10
7.5	12
8.0	12-14
8.5	12-14
9.0	14-16

Suction catheters should have the following characteristics:

Characteristic	Rationale
At least 20 cm in length	Allows catheter to pass the entire length of the ETT and slightly beyond, including through the tip
Molded ends: smooth, rounded, or ring tipped	Reduces trauma to the tracheobronchial mucosa
Multiple side holes	Reduces chance of invagination of tracheobronchial mucosa into suction catheter
Minimal friction resistance	Enhances ease of passing catheter through artificial airway
Proximal side vents; connectable to a Y adapter	Allows for intermittent application of suction
Suction control vent in opposite direction of suction flow	Reduces risk of contamination of hand regulating suction with secretions.
Sterile, disposable	Reduces risk of introducing bacteria into tracheobronchial tree

Closed suction system

Closed suction systems are available from multiple manufacturers. The advantages of a closed in-line system include continued oxygenation, reduction of loss of PEEP, decreased nursing time, decreased chance of aerolization of secretions, and decreased risk of introducing bacteria into the airway. These systems are beneficial in clients requiring high levels of PEEP and high FiO_2 and in those isolated for respiratory infections (Fig. 4-19). Specific recommendations for use of the closed suction system should be referred to the manufacturer. In-line suction systems are changed every 24 hours and changes should be coordinated with the changing of the ventilator circuit on patients receiving mechanical ventilation.

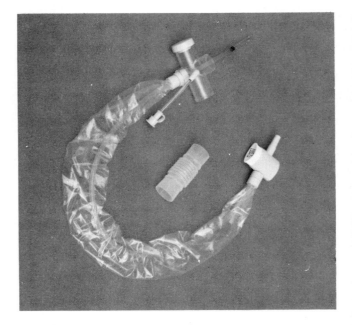

Figure 4-19
Closed suction system
(Courtesy Ballard Medical Products, Midvale, Utah.)

Chest Physiotherapy

Chest physiotherapy (CPT) includes the techniques of chest wall percussion, postural drainage (PD), and vibration and rib shaking to assist in the removal of tracheobronchial secretions. CPT is indicated in clients with bronchiectasis, infiltrates demonstrated on chest x-ray examinations, and sputum production of 30 ml per day or greater. Coupled with postural drainage, CPT provides effective pulmonary hygiene in the client whose mucociliary action has been impaired.

Percussion is performed by striking the chest wall with cupped hands (Fig. 4-20), generating a hollow, popping sound. Correctly performed, percussion is painless. Vibration is performed during exhalation using the flat part of the palm over the area treated. The client exhales through pursed lips while the clinician vibrates the area in the same direction as rib movement. Rib shaking also is performed during a prolonged exhalation through pursed lips. The ribs are rocked in a downward motion using the flat part of the hand. Rib shaking and vibration assist in dislodging mucous plugs. Percussion should be avoided over the spine, liver, kidney, abdomen, spleen, shoulder blades, and breast tissue. Contraindications for CPT/PD include hemoptysis, pulmonary emboli, osteoporosis, and bleeding disorders. Special precautions and/or modification of the procedure is indicated in acute myocardial infarction (MI), rib fracture, or flail chest, and following abdominal and thoracic surgery (see box).

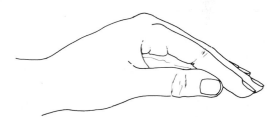

Figure 4-20
Cupped hand position
(From Wade JF: Comprehensive respiratory care, ed 3, St Louis, 1982, The CV Mosby Co.)

Special Considerations for CPT

Acute MI	Head down position may not be toler-
Hypotension	ated if CHF component is present
Hypertension	May cause headache
Rib fractures	Avoid clapping over suture line, area
Flail chest	of acute injury, or flail segment,
Thoracic surgery	since underlying tissue may be
	damaged. Premedicate the client
	with pain medication as indicated.
	Vibration may be more effective and
	less painful
Cerebral edema	Head down position will increase
Neurosurgery	intracranial pressure

Nursing considerations for CPT/PD are as follows:
1. Loosen tight clothing.
2. Be sure the client is comfortable and understands the procedure.
3. Perform vibration over a single layer of clothing or bath towel.
4. Clients may feel short of breath during postural drainage.
5. Periods of rest may be indicated.
6. Wait at least 1 hour after client has eaten to perform CPT.
7. Nasogastric small intestinal feedings should be held 1 hour before therapy.
8. Encourage deep breathing and coughing after therapy.
9. Provide suctioning if the client has difficulty removing secretions.

CPT/PD positions are as follows:

LOWER LOBES

Posterior basal segment	Elevate feet 30 degrees (Fig. 4-21)
	Prone position; 3 to 4 pillows under hips or head down
	Percuss/vibrate lower ribs

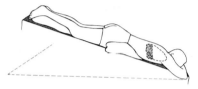

Figure 4-21

Lateral basal segment	Elevate feet 30 degrees, have client lie on side. Percuss and vibrate lower ribs(Fig. 4-22)

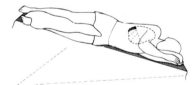

Figure 4-22

Superior segment	Have client lie on stomach with pillow under stomach (Fig. 4-23)
	Percuss/vibrate between shoulders and lower ribs.

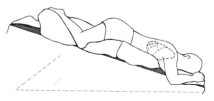

Figure 4-23

Anterior basal segment	Have client lie on back with knees flexed. Elevate foot of bed 30 degrees. Percuss/vibrate over lower ribs. (Fig. 4-24)

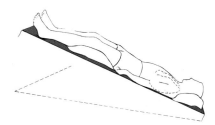

Figure 4-24

Right middle lobe (medial and lateral segments)	Have client lie on left side. (Fig. 4-25) Place pillow at back. Rotate ¼ turn back. Elevate foot of bed 15 degrees. Percuss/vibrate over nipple area

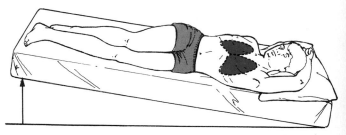

Figure 4-25

Lingula	Have client lie on right side. (Fig . 4-26)
	Place pillow at back.
	Rotate ¼ turn back.
	Elevate foot of bed 15 degrees.
	Percuss/vibrate over left nipple.

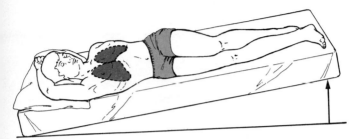

Figure 4-26

Upper Lobes

Anterior apical segment	Have client sit up in chair, then lean back. Percuss/vibrate at shoulders. Extend fingers over collarbone. (Fig. 4-27)

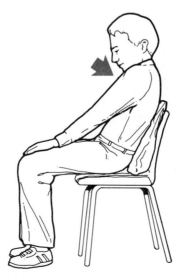

Figure 4-27

Posterior apical segment — Have client sit up in chair, then lean forward over pillow. Percuss/vibrate at shoulders. (Fig. 4-28)

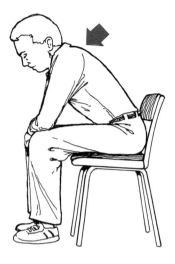

Figure 4-28

Left upper lobe posterior segment — Have client lie on right side, then rotate forward, leaning over pillow. Percuss/vibrate over left shoulder. (Fig. 4-29)

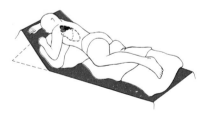

Figure 4-29

| Right upper lobe posterior segment | Have client lie on left side, rotating ¼ turn forward onto pillow for support. (Fig. 4-30) Bed should be flat. Percuss/vibrate over right shoulder blade. |

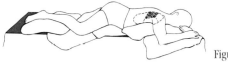

Figure 4-30

| Anterior segment | Have client lie flat on back. Percuss/vibrate just below collarbone. (Fig. 4-31) |

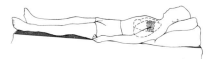

Figure 4-31

Emergency Management
Airway obstruction

The initial assessment step of any emergency situation is to establish airway patency. The tongue is the most frequent cause of airway obstruction in the unconscious client. Opening the airway with the chin lift/jaw thrust technique is recommended. If head and neck trauma is suspected, the chin lift/jaw-thrust technique is applied. (AHA, 1987). If the airway remains obstructed after positioning the head, obstructed airway maneuvers are indicated. Abdominal thrusts are administered while straddling the client in an attempt to dislodge the obstruction. It is imperative to continue to relieve an airway obstruction until successful or until emergency surgical intervention such as cricothyroid stick or emergency tracheostomy can be implemented.

Airway obstruction in the conscious client requires assessment of the degree of obstruction. Partial obstruction requires support of the client and continued observation for progression to complete obstruction. Complete airway obstruction is indicated by inability to speak and no movement of air and requires immediate intervention. Abdominal thrusts are administered from behind the client, who should be continually assessed for relief of obstruction. If the client loses consciousness, he or she should be eased to the floor and reassessed for breathing. If the obstruction continues, abdominal thrusts as described previously should be administered.

Esophageal obturator

The esophageal obturator airway (EOA) is a large-diameter airway with an occluded distal end (Fig. 4-31). The tube, when correctly positioned, has many ventilation ports that lie in the posterior pharynx. The tube measures 37 cm in length, and a large 35 ml balloon is at the distal end. When positioned correctly and inflated, the balloon prevents positive pressure ventilation from inflating the stomach and causing regurgitation of gastric contents. A clear mask is connected to the EOA tube. When the mask is fitted properly, ventilation is delivered through the EOA to the lungs (Fig. 4-32).

EOAs are most often used in emergency medical systems (EMS) by paramedics as an alternative to endotracheal intubation (Fig. 4-33). EOAs should be inserted by clinicians who have been properly trained and have become proficient in their use (AHA, 1987).

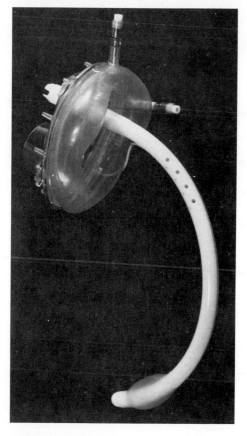

Figure 4-32
Esophageal obturator airway.
(From Sheehy S: Emergency nursing, St Louis, 1985, The CV Mosby Co). Photo
by Richard Lazar.

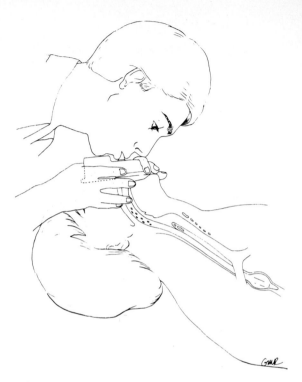

Figure 4-33
Esophageal obturator airway in place.
(From Sheehy S: Manual of emergency care, ed 3, St Louis, 1990, The CV
Mosby Co.)

Insertion techniques are as follows:
1. Attach mask to tube.
2. Check balloon for patency.
3. Deflate cuff completely.
4. Lubricate the tube.
5. Position the head in midposition or slight flexion.
6. Lift the tongue and jaw with nondominant hand.
7. Insert tube through mouth into esophagus.
8. Advance tube until mask is seated on the face.
9. Administer positive pressure ventilation before inflating the cuff.
10. Observe for chest rise and fall.
11. Inflate balloon slowly with 35 cc air.
12. Auscultate the lungs bilaterally for breath sounds.
13. Auscultate the epigastrium for gurgling, which indicates that the tube is incorrectly placed.

Nursing Considerations	Rationale
Remove EOA after 2 hours and provide tracheal intubation	Reduces chance of esophageal necrosis from inflated cuff
Suction should be readily available during removal	Most clients will vomit after removal of the EOA
Before tube removal the client should be positioned on the side or with the head turned to the side	Facilitates the removal of gastric secretions
ETT should be in place before removing the EOA	Protects the airway from aspiration

Endotracheal intubation

Preferably, endotracheal intubation is an elective procedure based on clinical assessment of secretion management and/or respiratory failure. However, intubation of the trachea does occur frequently in emergent situations such as cardiopulmonary arrest, anaphylatic reactions, and trauma. The most common reason for endotracheal intubation is initiation of mechanical ventilation (Trulock and Schuster, 1986). Intubation is also indicated for airway protection and pulmonary hygiene.

Endotracheal intubation should be performed by a skilled clinician. Direct laryngoscopic intubation technique is recommended in the emergent situation.

Step	Nursing Considerations
Gather intubation equipment	May be located in an intubation tray or an emergency cart
	ETT sizes 6.0-10.0 mm
	Laryngoscope handle
	Batteries
	Extra light bulbs
	Laryngoscope bladers—curved, straight
	Water-soluble lubricant
	Stylet
	Towel
	Tape
	McGill forceps
	10 ml syringe
	Suction equipment
Assemble laryngoscope	Check to be sure that the light is working
Select size and check ETT for function	Females: 7.0-8.0 mm
	Males: 8.0-8.5 mm
	Maintaining sterility of the ETT; check the cuff for integrity
Prepare the ETT	Lubricate with sterile water-soluble lubricant
Position client	Lie supine with head extended and neck flexed "sniffing position"). The towel may be used under the head to help elevate it slightly
Clear oral airway	Suction immediately before intubation

Step	Nursing Considerations
Intubation	Assist as indicated. Have suction ready. Auscultate for breath sounds bilaterally after the tube has been placed. Secure ETT in place
Obtain chest x-ray examination	Determines ETT placement; requires physician's order

During the preparation time it is imperative that the client is adequately ventilated. An oral airway may be indicated to maintain airway patency. If an intubation attempt is not successful after 30 seconds, it should be stopped and ventilation resumed. The clinician should continuously assess the client for heart rate and rhythm, especially bradycardia secondary to vagal response, color, and tolerance of the procedure. Ressure the client throughout the procedure.

Complications of endotracheal intubation are as follows:
Intubation of right mainstem bronchus
Intubation of the esophagus
Laceration of the lips and gums
Broken teeth
Pharyngeal laceration
Oral-pharyngeal bleeding
Damage to the vocal cords
Aspiration
Hypoxia

Cricothyroid stick/cricothyrotomy

The cricothyroid stick is accomplished by inserting a catheter-over-needle large-bore catheter through the cricothyroid membrane for airway access. Cricothyrotomy is the opening of the cricothyroid membrane with a scapel for rapid access to the airway. Complete obstruction of the upper airway is the most frequent indication for these techniques. Both procedures are usually physician responsibilities in acute care settings. Nursing responsibilities include assisting the physician; monitoring vital signs; assisting the client; and observing for complications such as bleeding, hematoma, and subcutaneous emphysema (Fig. 4-34).

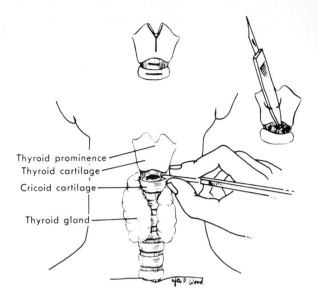

Figure 4-34
Criothyrotomy incision.
(From Miller RH and Cantrell JR: Textbook of basic medicine, St Louis, 1975,
The CV Mosby Co.)

Emergency tracheostomy

Surgical opening of the trachea and placement of a tracheostomy
tube should ideally be performed in the operating room (AHA,
1987). If this is not possible, the nurse's responsibilities lie in assisting the physician during the procedure:

1. Obtain:
   a. Tracheostomy insertion tray
   b. Sterile gloves
   c. Local anesthetic
   d. Suture: 4-0 silk and 3-0 silk
   e. Tracheostomy tube and tracheostomy care kit

2. Assemble suction equipment
3. Reassure client as necessary
4. Obtain baseline data: BP, pulse, heart rhythm, respiratory pattern
5. Assist physician as indicated

References

Ackerman MH: The use of bolus normal saline instillations in artificial airways: is it useful or necessary? Heart Lung 14(5):505, 1985.

American Heart Association: Adjuncts for airway control, ventilation and supplemental oxygen. In Textbook of advanced cardiac life support, Dallas, 1987, The Association.

Holloway NM: Acute aeriation disorders in nursing the critically ill adult, Reading, ed 3, 1988, Addison-Wesley Publishing Co Inc.

Perry A and Potter P: Clinical nursing skills and techniques, ed 2, St. Louis, Mosby–Year Book Inc.

Trulock EP and Schuster DP: Acute respiratory failure. In The manual of medical therapeutics, Boston, 1986, Little, Brown, & Co, Inc.

Zschoche DA, editor: Mosby's comprehensive review of critical care, ed 3, St Louis, 1985, The CV Mosby Co.

Bibliography

Chulay M and Graeber GM: Efficacy of hyperinflation and hyperoxygenation after suctioning intervention, Heart Lung 17(1):15, 1988.

Goodenough SK: Reducing tracheal injury and aspiration, Dim Crit Care Nurs 7(6):324, 1988.

Harper RW: Management of airways. In A guide to respiratory care physiology and clinical applications, Philadelphia, 1981, JB Lippincott Co.

Kluber C, Krutzfield N, and Rose E: Acute histologic changes in the tracheobronchial tree associated with different suction catheter insertion techniques, Heart Lung 17(1):10, 1988.

Mayhall CG: The trach care closed tracheal suction system: a new medical device to permit tracheal suctioning without interruption of ventilatory assistance, Infect Control Hosp Epidemiol 9(3):125, 1988.

McHugh J: Perfecting the three steps of chest physiotherapy, Nursing 87, November.

Preusser BA et al: Effects of two methods of preoxygenation on mean arterial pressure, cardiac output, peak airway pressure, and post suctioning hypoxemia. Heart Lung 17(3):290, 1988.

Shapiro BA, Harrison RA, and Trent CA: Clinical application of respiratory care, ed 3, Chicago, 1985, Yearbook Medical Publishers.

Springhouse Corporation: Clinical pocket manual of respiratory care, Springhouse, Pennsylvania, 1985.

Springhouse Corporation: Respiratory care handbook, Springhouse Corporation, Springhouse, Pennsylvania, 1989.

Travers GA: Respiratory nursing: the science and the art, New York, 1982, John Wiley & Sons, Inc.

Zadar C: Chest physical therapy. In Morrison ML, editor: Respiratory intensive care nursing, Boston, 1979, Little, Brown & Co, Inc.

Respiratory Medications

5

Bronchodilators

Bronchodilators are used to relieve bronchospasm in asthma, acute and chronic bronchitis, and status asthmaticus. Bronchodilators are divided into two categories: the sympathomimetic agents and the methyl xanthine agents. The most common side effects of bronchodilators include feelings of nervousness, increase in heart rate, tremor, and palpitations (see box).

Side Effects of Bronchodilators

Tachycardia	Flushing
Tremor	Increased blood pressure
Nervousness	Headache
Palpitations	Nausea
Dizziness	Vomiting
Sweating	Restlessness
Arrhythmias	Irritability
Difficulty sleeping	

Sympathomimetics

Sympathomimetics (adrenergic) bronchodilators act by stimulating the beta$_2$ receptors in the lung resulting in bronchial smooth muscle relaxation and reduction of bronchial secretions. Sympathomimetics also have alpha and beta$_1$ effects. The alpha effects include vasoconstriction and increase in blood pressure. Inhaled bronchodilators with alpha effects produce a decrease in bronchial congestion and an increase in the duration of action for beta$_2$ bronchodilators when given together (Karb et al., 1989). The beta$_1$ effects are cardiac specific and include increased heart rate, increased force of myocardial contraction, and increased rate of repolarization (Karb et al., 1989). Sympathomimetic agents should be used with caution in elderly clients and those with heart disease. Doses should be adjusted downward to prevent side effects. Abuse of inhaled sympathomimetics can result in worsening of bronchospasm in some clients. The effects of the beta$_2$ stimulating bronchodilators are inhibited by the concomitant administration of beta-adrenergic blocking agents. Prolonged use of sympathomimetics can result in development of a tolerance to the effects of the medication.

Drug	Dosage	Nursing Considerations
Albuterol sulfate (Proventil, Ventolin)	Metered dose inhaler (MDI): 1-2 puffs q 4-6 hr	May cause paradoxical bronchoconstriction
	By mouth (PO): 1-2 mg q 4-6 hr	
	Nebulized: 2.5 mg in 2.5 ml NS q 4-6 hr	
Ephedrine sulfate (Ectasule Minus)	PO: 25-50 mg q 3-4 hr	Elderly clients are more sensitive to the drug
	Extended release preparation: 15, 30, or 60 mg q 8-12 hr	Monitor mental status

Drug	Dosage	Nursing Considerations
	For severe broncho-spasm: IM or SC: 12.5-25 mg	
Epinephrine (Adren-alin)	IM or SC: (1:1000) 0.2-0.5 mg q 20 min to 4 hr as needed	Use TB syringe to draw up medica-tion; do not ad-minister in conjunction with Isuprel
		Monitor vital signs for increased heart rate and blood pressure
Epinephrine (race-mic) (Vaponefrin, MicroNEFRIN 2.25%)	Inhalation: aerosol nebulizers deliver 0.2 mg per inha-lation	Allow 1-2 minutes between inhala-tions
Epinephrine bitar-trate (Asthma Meter, Medihaler-Epi, Primatene Mist)	Inhalation: aerosol nebulizer delivers 0.2 mg per inha-lation. Medihaler-Epi de-livers 0.1 mg per inhalation	Available over-the-counter Inform client not to use over-the-counter drugs without consult-ing a physician
Epinephrine suspen-sion (Sus-Phrine)	SC:0.1-0.3 mg q 6 hr	Mix vial or ampule well by shaking. Draw up and ad-minister immedi-ately. Use TB syringe
Isoetharine (Bronko-sol)	Inhalation: 3-7 in-halations by hand nebulizer IPPB: 0.25-1 ml in 3 ml NS	Do not exceed 12 inhalations per day Allow 1 minute between inhala-tions

Drug	Dosage	Nursing Considerations
Isoetharine mesylate (Bronkometer)	Inhalation— aerosol: 1-4 inhalations q 3-6 hr	Do not exceed 12 inhalations per 24 hours
Isoproterenol (Isuprel) Isuprel Mistometer, Isuprel Elixir)	Inhalation— Mistometer 6-8 inhalations q 3 hr PO: Elixer 2 tbsp 3-4 times/day	Should not be given in conjunction with epinephrine Allow 1-5 minutes between inhalations
Metaproterenol sulfate (Alupent, Metaprel)	PO: 10 mg 3-4 times/day Increase to 20 mg 3-4 times/day over 2-4 weeks Inhalation—MDI: 2-3 inhalations q 3-4 hr	Do not exceed 12 inhalations in 24 hours Allow 2 minutes between inhalations Should precede steroid inhalation (when prescribed) by 15 minutes for maximal benefit
Terbutaline (Brethine, Bricanyl)	PO: 5 mg 3 times daily SC: 0.25 mg; may be repeated in 15-30 minutes	Do not exceed 15 mg in 24 hours Beta blockers may inhibit effects No more than 0.5 mg in 4-hour period

Drug	Dosage	Nursing Considerations
	Inhalation—Bretine MDI: 2 inhalations every 4-6 hr	Wait 1 minute between inhalations (10-20 minutes between inhalations is suggested)
		Do not give with MAO inhibitors, since interaction may lead to hypertensive crisis
		If paradoxical bronchospasm develops, discontinue drug immediately

Methylxanthines

Methylxanthines promote bronchodilatation by relaxing bronchial smooth muscle. Other effects include cardiac muscle stimulation, central nervous system stimulation, and diuresis. Patients who smoke require larger doses of methylxanthines because the half-life of the drug is reduced.

Methylxanthines have a narrow range of therapeutic blood levels. Clients should be monitored closely for side effects of nausea, tachycardia, palpitations, and nervousness. Therapy should be guided by periodic checks of blood levels. Desired serum theophylline levels are 10-20 μg/ml (Karb et al., 1989). Theophylline and aminophylline are not equivalent on a one-to-one basis. Theophylline 20 mg is equal to aminophylline 25 mg.

Drug	Dosage	Nursing Considerations
Aminophylline (Theophylline ethylenediamine)	IV: diluted to 25 mg/ml Loading dose: 5.6 mg/kg over 30 min Maintenance dose: 0.3-0.9 mg/kg/hr continuous IV infusion	Do not administer faster than 25 mg/min; IV administration should be given by volumetric pump. Rapid IV administration can cause tachycardia and cardiovascular collapse
	Rectal: 250-500 mg 1-3 times/ day PO: Acute — 500 mg followed by maintenance dose: 200-250 mg q 6-8 hr	Refrigerate suppositories Give with food to reduce GI irritation
Dyphylline (Dilin, Dilor Dyflex, Emgabid, Lufyllin, Neothyllin)	PO: 200-800 mg q 6 hr IM: 250-500 mg	*See* Aminophylline IV use not recommended; metabolized faster than theophylline; may need increased dose
Oxtriphylline (Choledyl, Theolair, Theolair SR, Theophyl SR)	PO: 200 mg q 6 hr	*See* Aminophylline Protect from light and store at 15°-30° C

Drug	Dosage	Nursing Considerations
Theophylline (Theo-Dur, Elixophyllin, Ourbren, Slophyllin, Bronkodyl)	PO: Initial dose 3-5 mg/kg q 6 hr Maintenance 100-200 mg q 6 hr	*See* Aminophylline May cause dizziness in elderly clients
	Rectal: 250-500 mg q 8-12 hr	Keep refrigerated

Anticholinergics

Anticholinergics block the action of the vagus nerve, thereby decreasing airway secretions and preventing or reversing bronchoconstriction.

Drug	Dosage	Nursing Considerations
Atropine sulfate	Inhalation— nebulized: 0.025 mg/kg in 3-5 ml NS 3-4 times/day	Do not exceed 2.5 mg/dose May cause drying of secretions
Ipratropium bromide (Atrovent)	Inhalation: 2 inhalations 4 times a day	Do not exceed 12 inhalations in 24 hours. When using another MDI bronchodilator, use the Atrovent second. Atrovent does not have rapid reversal of bronchospasm and is not indicated for acute attacks

Corticosteroids

Corticosteroids are used to reduce inflammation of the bronchial mucosa and to stabilize cell walls thereby preventing the release of hydrolytic enzymes. The clinician must be aware of the many side effects and precautions when administering long-term steroid therapy (see box). These include changes in mood and behavior, development of diabetes, sodium retention and potassium loss, increased susceptibility to infection, osteoporosis or bone fractures, peptic ulcer or gastric irritation, and development of a moon face. Many clients have an increase in appetite. Prolonged use is also associated with fat deposits on the trunk of the body.

Side Effects of Corticosteroids

Central Nervous System	Anxiety
	Depression
	Euphoria
	Insomnia
	Mood swings
	Increased motor activity
Cardiovascular	Fluid retention
	Congestive heart failure
	Thromboembolic disease
	Palpitations
	Thrombocytopenia
Skin	Bruising
	Acne
	Atrophy of the skin
	Facial erythema
Musculoskeletal	Muscle pain
	Weakness
	Muscle wasting
	Delayed wound healing
	Fractures
Endocrine	Decreased glucose tolerance
	Hyperglycemia
	Aggravation of diabetes mellitus

(Adapted from Karb VB, Queener SF, and Freeman JB: Handbook of drugs for nursing practice, pp 603-605, 1989, St. Louis, The CV Mosby Co.)

Drug	Dosage	Nursing Considerations
Beclomethasone dipropionate (Beclovent, Vanceril)	Inhalation: 2 inhalations 3-4 times/day. Each inhalation is 42 μg. Daily dose should not exceed 840 μg (20 inhalations)	Have client rinse mouth after use to prevent oral candidal infection
Flunisolide (Aero-Bid, Nasalide)	Inhalation—intranasal: 2 inhalations (50 μg) twice daily Oral: initially 2 inhalations (500 μg) every AM and PM. Not to exceed 2000 μg/day	Have client rinse mouth after use to prevent oral candidal infection Oral inhalation may relieve symptoms of bronchial asthma Onset of effect may take 1-4 weeks to develop (Karb et al., 1989)
Triamcinalone acetonide (Azmacort)	Inhalation—MDI: 2 inhalations 3-4 times/day	Have client rinse mouth after use
Prednisone (Meticorten, Orasone)	PO: 5-60 mg daily given in 2-4 doses/day	Preferable to give in AM Give with food
Hydrocortisone (Cortef) Hydrocortisone phosphate Hydrocortisone succinate	PO: 5-30 mg 3-4 times/day IM: Initial dose 100-250 mg (succinate), then 50-100 mg IM as indicated	Give oral dosage with food

Drug	Dosage	Nursing Considerations
	IV: 100-250 mg (succinate) initially; 15-240 mg (phosphate) q 12 hr	

Cromolyn Sodium

Cromolyn sodium is a drug used in the treatment of asthma. Cromolyn is given to stabilize the mast cells to prevent degranulation and release of bronchospastic mediators (Karb et al., 1989). Cromolyn is not indicated for the relief of an acute asthmatic attack, but rather it is given prophylactically. Side effects include dizziness, drowsiness, and headache. Gastrointestinal side effects include nausea and stomach ache. Upon initial administration of cromolyn, the client should be monitored for wheezing, bronchospasm, sneezing, and irritation of the throat.

Drug	Dosage	Nursing Considerations
Cromolyn sodium (Intal)	Inhalation: 20 mg capsule 4 times/ day	No effect in acute attacks
		May cause irritation of the throat
		GI side effects can be reduced by advising milk intake before client takes medication
		Medication can be inhaled into the lungs via the mouth or nose

Expectorants

Expectorants are used to thin the fluid and increase the output of fluid from the respiratory tract. Increasing oral fluid intake is an effective way to thin and liquify respiratory secretions.

Drug	Dosage	Nursing Considerations
Potassium iodide (SSKI, Potassium Iodide)	PO: 300 mg q 4-6 hr	Dilute in large amount of fluid
		Give after meals
		Do not give to clients with iodide sensitivity, tuberculosis, hyperkalemia, acute bronchitis, or hyperthyroidism
Guaifenesin (glycerol guaiacolate) (Antituss, Robitussin)	Dosage PO: 100-200 mg q 3-4 hr	Watch for bleeding gums and bruising in clients also taking heparin
		May cause nausea
		Available over-the-counter
Iodinated glycerol (organidin)	PO: 20 drops (50 mg) or 60 mg tablet or 5 ml elixir (60 mg) 4 times/day	Do not give to clients with iodine sensitivity

Mucolytic Agents

Mucolytic agents reduce the thickness of sputum, thereby increasing the ease of sputum production. Mucolytics break down the mucoproteins of respiratory secretions into smaller, less viscous strands (Hahn et al, 1982). Aerosol administration is the usual route. Fifteen to 30 minutes after an aerosol treatment, the clinician must be alert for an outpouring of respiratory secretions and provide adequate pulmonary hygiene measures such as tracheal suctioning, facial tissues, and support during periods of coughing and expectoration.

Drug	Dosage	Nursing Considerations
Acetylcysteine (Mucomyst)	Inhalation— nebulized: 1-10 ml of 20% solution or 2-20 ml of a 10% solution q 2-6 hr	Be prepared for marked increase in sputum production 15-20 minutes after treatment
		Discontinue for bronchospasm in asthmatics

Antitussives

Antitussives are cough suppressants that suppress the cough reflex in the medullary center. Cough suppressives are indicated for symptomatic relief. Central nervous system depression including respiratory depression, stupor, and coma can result when antitussives with opiate or antihistamines are combined with other CNS depressants (Karb et al., 1989).

Drug	Dosage	Nursing Considerations
Codeine	PO: 10-20 mg q 4-6 hr	Effects seen in 1-2 hours; duration of action is 4 hours.
		Monitor client for mood changes, dizziness, sedation, heart rate and BP changes
		Do not exceed 120 mg in 24 hours
Diphenhydramine hydrochloride (Benylin)	PO: 25 mg q 4 hr	No more than 100 mg in 24 hours
		May cause drowsiness

Antitubergularis Drugs

The drugs in this section are used specifically to treat persons with *Mycobacterium tuberculosis* or those who have been exposed to active disease. It is important that the client and family be educated about tuberculosis and encouraged to continue the medical regime and follow-up care.

Drug	Dosage	Nursing Considerations
Ethambutol hydro-chloride (Etibi, Myambutol)	Initial treatment— PO: 15 mg/kg daily Retreatment— PO: 25 mg/kg daily x 60 days; decrease to 15 mg/kg daily	Should not be used alone Second antitubercular drug is also given Monitor for decreased vision during therapy Dosage is decreased in renal disease Hepatic, renal, and hemolytic parameters are monitored
Isoniazid (INH)	Primary therapy— PO: 5 mg/kg daily up to 300 mg/day IM: same as PO	Therapy lasts for 9-12 months Should not be given alone to treat tuberculosis Instruct client to avoid alcoholic beverages
Rifampin (Rifaden, Rofact)	PO: 600 mg daily	Give 1 hour before or 2 hours after meal Monitor hepatic function

Drug	Dosage	Nursing Considerations
		Urine may become red-orange color.
		Instruct client to avoid alcoholic beverages
		Usually used with one other drug
Streptomycin sulfate	Normal renal function: IM: 1 g (or 15 mg/kg) daily then 1 g 2-3 times/week	Given for 2-3 months
		Deep IM injection
		Use upper outer quadrant of the buttocks.
		Monitor renal function
		Use with at least one other antituberculosis drug

Antifungals/Antiprotozoals

Antifungal and antiprotozoal drugs are used to treat infections caused by fungi and protozoas.

Drug	Dosage	Nursing Considerations
Amphotericin B	Initial test dose: IV: 1 mg/250 ml D$_5$W over 2-4 hr Maintenance dose: 0.25 mg/kg/day over 6 hr Range .25-.50 mg/kg/day	Do not exceed 1.5 mg/kg/day May develop fever 1-2 hours after infusion starts. May be premedicated with acetaminophen and benadryl as ordered

Drug	Dosage	Nursing Considerations
		Monitor for potassium depletion
		Check liver and renal functions and CBC weekly
Ketoconazole	PO: 200 mg daily; may be increased to 400 mg daily	Use with caution in clients with diminished liver function
Miconazole	IV: 200-3600 mg/day. Given in 3 divided doses	Dilute in at least 200 ml NS
		Rapid infusion may produce arrhythmias
		Give IV for a period of 30-60 minutes
Pentamidine isethionate	IV: 4 mg/kg daily for 14 days	May develop hypotension.
	IM: 4 mg/kg daily for 14 days	Infuse for a period of 60 minutes
	Inhalation: 30-300 mg dissolved in 6 ml sterile water	Treatment times vary from 30-45 minutes
		During inhalation instruct patient to breathe deeply and inhale and exhale through the mouth
		Used with Respirgard II nebulizer system

Drug Used in Treatment of Infections of Fungi and Protozoas

Amphotericin	Histoplasmosis
	Coccidioidomycosis
	Crytococcosis
	Aspergillosis
	Phycomycosis
Ketoconazole	Candidiasis
	Histoplasmosis
Miconazole	Systemic candidiasis
	Paracoccidioidomycosis
	Cryptococcosis
Pentamidine isethionate	Pneumocystis carinii

Drugs Used During Intubation and Mechanical Ventilation

Drugs used during intubation and mechanical ventilation should be used with caution. The medications result in respiratory muscle paralysis or in depression of respiratory drive. It is important to monitor the client frequently; assess vital signs including respiratory rate, pattern, and drive; and provide adequate mechanical ventilation for those drugs resulting in respiratory muscle depression or paralysis. Those medications causing respiratory muscle paralysis do not provide sedation in many clients. It is important for the clinician to provide additional sedation for the client, as well as emotional support to the client and his or her family. Being paralyzed and unable to communicate, yet being able to hear and see, is very frightening for the client. These drugs are usually given in the intensive care unit setting; however, they may be used on a general nursing care division during an emergent situation such as emergent intubation.

Drug	Dosage	Nursing Considerations
Pancuronium bromide (Pavulon)	IV: 0.04-0.1 mg/kg, then 0.01 mg/kg q 30-60 min as needed	Refrigerate drug Monitor client closely Provide mechanical ventilation If client is still awake and alert, consider sedation Provide eye drops to keep eyes moist Antidote: Neostigmine (refrigerate drug)
Succinylcholine chloride (Anectine)	IV: 25-75 mg, then 2.5 mg/min IM: 2.5 mg/kg	Monitor client closely Client must be mechanically ventilated If client is still awake and alert, consider sedation Provide eye drops to keep eyes moist Maximum dosage: 150 mg If given IM, use the deltoid muscle Refrigerate drug
Diazepam (Valium)	IV: 1-2 mg over 5-10 min	Give slow IV push Administer close to venipuncture site

Drug	Dosage	Nursing Considerations
Morphine sulfate	IV: 2.5 mg-16 mg diluted in 5 ml saline	Give slow IV push
		Monitor client slowly for hypotension and respiratory depression
		Antidote: Narcon

Respiratory Stimulant

A respiratory stimulant is used in clients with depressed respiration caused by a drug overdose or COPD. Although they are used infrequently, they are available.

Drug	Dosage	Nursing Considerations
Dorapram hydrochloride (Dopram)	IV: 0.5-1.0 mg/kg Infusion: 1-3 mg/min	Maximum dose: 4 mg/kg up to 3 g/day
	COPD infusion: 1-2 mg/min	Maximum dose: 3 mg/min up to 2 hours of infusion
		Monitor vital signs continuously during administration and for 30-60 minutes afterward
		Maintain a patent airway
		Have O_2 and intubation equipment available
		Narrow safety margin

References

Hahn AB, Barkin RL, and Oestreich SJK: Pharmacology in nursing, ed 15, St Louis, 1982, The CV Mosby Co.

Karb VB, Queener SF, and Freeman JB: Handbook of drugs for nursing practice, St Louis, 1989, The CV Mosby Co.

Bibliography

Boehringer Ingelheim: Atrovent (ipiatropium bromide) inhalation aerosol, 1987, Ridgefield, Connecticut, Boehringer Ingelheim.

Clark JB, Queener SF, and Karb VB: Pharmacological basis of nursing practice, St Louis, 1982, The CV Mosby Co.

Clark JB, Queener SF, and Karb VB: Pocket nurse guide to drugs, St Louis, 1986, The CV Mosby Co.

Clayton BD: Mosby's handbook of pharmacology in nursing, ed 4, St Louis, 1987, The CV Mosby Co.

Grass NJ and Skorodin MS: State of the art anticholinergic, antimuscarinic bronchodilators, Am Rev Respir Dis 129:856-870, 1984.

Habib MP et al: A comparison of albuterol and metaproterenol nebulizer solutions, Ann Allergy 58(6):421, 1987.

Montgomery AB et al: Aerosolised pentamidine as sole therapy for pneumocystis carinii pneumonia in patients with acquired immunodeficiency syndrome, Lancet, August 29, 1987.

Nursing 88: New hope for AIDS patients with pneumocystis pneumonia, Nursing 88, February.

Petty TL: Drug strategies for airflow obstruction, Am J Nurs February 1987.

Springhouse Corporation: Respiratory care handbook, Springhouse, Pennsylvania, 1989, Springhouse Corporation.

Oxygenation

6

Indications for supplemental oxygen use are as follows:

Hypoxemia (low Pao_2)

Increased myocardial work

Decreased cardiac output

Increased work of breathing

Increased oxygen demand

Sepsis

Infection

Decreased oxygen carrying capacity

Carbon monoxide poisoning

Sickle Cell Disease

When oxygen is in use, several safety procedures must be followed:

- Keep oxygen source 10 feet from open flame
- Do not use electrical appliances within 5 feet of oxygen source
- Do not use creams, oils, or petroleum-based products around oxygen system
- Secure oxygen system away from heat or direct sunlight
- No smoking in room with oxygen system
- Notify the fire department of home oxygen system
- Turn the oxygen off when not in use

Oxygen Delivery Systems
Low-Flow Systems

A low-flow oxygen delivery system does not meet the entire inspiratory requirements of the client. Room air is entrained by the client during inspiration. Dilution of the inspired flow is dependent on the depth and rate of the inspiratory effort. Low-flow systems provide approximate levels of oxygen.

Low-flow systems are used with more stable clients. They are easy to apply and more comfortable for the client to wear.

Nasal cannula (Fig. 6-1)

Indications	Advantages/ Disadvantages	Nursing Considerations
COPD	Disposable	Nares need to be patent
Paco$_2$ retainers	Easy to apply	
	Comfortable	Maintain humidification for liter flow >4 liter per minutes (LPM)
	Inexpensive	
	Cannot control O$_2$ concentration	Give oral/nasal care every 8 hr
	Dries and irritates nasal mucosa	Observe for pressure sores over ears and under nose
		When used in patients with COPD, the liter flow is 1-4 LPM guided by the Paco$_2$

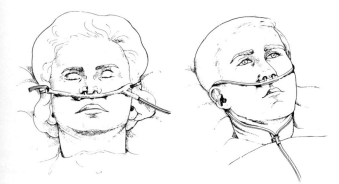

Figure 6-1
Nasal cannula
(From Wade JF: Comprehensive respiratory care, ed 3, St Louis, 1982, The CV Mosby Co.)

Approximate Fio_2 with Nasal Cannula

1L	24%
2L	28%
3L	32%
4L	36%
5L	40%
6L	44%

Simple face mask (Fig. 6-2)

Indications	Advantages/ Disadvantages	Nursing Considerations
Moderate hypoxemia	Well tolerated in adults	Recommend flow rate 8-10 LPM to provide 40%-60% Fio_2
Oxygen needs of >40% Fio_2	Does not dry mucous membranes because of humidification	
Short-term administration		Clean face every 2-3 hours
	Tight seal may be uncomfortable to some clients	Observe for pressure sores along edge of mask
	May irritate the skin	Some clients feel the need to remove the mask to communicate
	Cannot wear while eating	
	Not recommended for clients with COPD	Instruct the client in the importance of wearing mask correctly

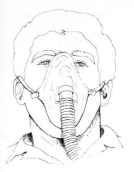

Figure 6-2
Simple face mask
(From Abels LF: Mosby's manual of critical care, St Louis, 1979, The CV Mosby Co.)

Approximate Fio_2 for Face Mask

5-6 LPM	40%
6-7 LPM	50%
7-8 LPM	60%

Face tent (Fig. 6-3)

Indications	Advantages/ Disadvantages	Nursing Considerations
Moderate hypoxemia	High humidity system helps to liquify secretions Less confining	Flow rate of 8-10 LPM delivers approximately 40% Fio_2
	Oxygen concentration cannot be controlled	Observe face/chin for signs of pressure sores
	May be irritating Must be removed to eat	Remove mask every 2-3 hours and clean face
	Can easily slip out of place	

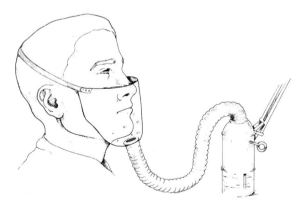

Figure 6-3
Face tent
(From Abels LF: Mosby's manual of critical care, St Louis, 1979, The CV Mosby Co.)

Partial rebreathing mask (Fig. 6-4)

Indications	Advantages/ Disadvantages	Nursing Considerations
Moderate to severe hypoxia	Humidified	6 LPM provides approximately 60% FiO_2
	Does not dry mucous membranes	Flow increases of 1 LPM increases FiO_2 by approximately 10%
	Mask may be uncomfortable and confining	Observe the reservoir bag during inspiration; it should not collapse completely
	Mask must fit snugly to ensure tight seal	Collapsing bags indicate a need for a higher flow rate
		Remove mask every 2-3 hours and clean face

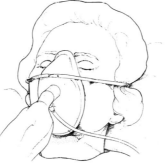

Figure 6-4
Partial rebreathing mask
(From Abels LF: Mosby's manual of critical care, St Louis, 1979, The CV Mosby Co.)

Nonrebreather mask (Fig. 6-5)

Indications	Advantages/ Disadvantages	Nursing Considerations
Severe hypoxia	Provides humidification	Provides Fio_2 of 60%-90%
Short-term therapy	Does not dry nasal/ oral mucosa	Observe reservoir bag to ensure that it does not totally deflate with inspiration
	Requires tight seal of face mask	Observe face for signs of pressure sores
	May be uncomfortable and confining	Observe client to ensure that flaps do not stick and prevent inhalation/ exhalation
		Remove mask every 2-3 hours and clean face
		Contraindicated in clients with COPD and CO_2 retention because of high O_2 concentration

Figure 6-5
Nonrebreathing mask
(From Abels LF: Mosby's manual of critical care, St Louis, 1979, The CV Mosby Co.)

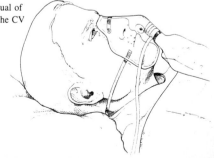

Tracheostomy collar (Fig. 6-6)

Indications	Advantages/ Disadvantages	Nursing Considerations
Provides high humidity and oxygen to client with tracheostomy	High humidity Frontal suctioning port Easily applied and removed Comfortable for client Helps keep secretions thinned Secretions can accumulate in tracheostomy collar	Clean tracheostomy collar every 3-4 hours Drain excess water from tubing frequently

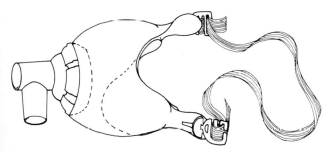

Figure 6-6
Tracheostomy collar
(From Wade JF: Comprehensive respiratory care, ed 3, St Louis, 1982, The CV Mosby Co.)

T piece (Fig. 6-7)

Indications	Advantages/ Disadvantages	Nursing Considerations
Provides high humidity and oxygen to client with ETT or tracheostomy	Increased client mobility	Clean T piece every 2-3 hours
	Easily applied	Drain excess water from tubing frequently
	Humidification	Usually has 6-inch piece of tubing attached to exhalation side to help regulate Fio_2 by decreasing room air entrainment
	Helps keep secretions thinned	
	Comfortable	
	Secretions easily accumulate in adaptor	
	May adhere to ETT/ tracheostomy from humidity/ secretions	Set-up can be adapted to create a high-flow system
		Monitor clients closely for accumulation of secretions and need for frequent suctioning

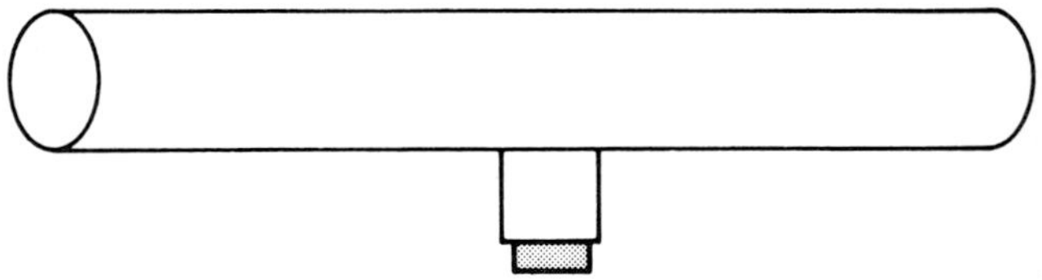

Figure 6-7
T-piece
(From Wade JF: Comprehensive respiratory care, ed 3, St Louis, 1982, The CV Mosby Co.)

High-Flow System

A high-flow delivery system is one in which the client's total inspiratory demands are provided. This system allows precise delivery of a specific oxygen concentration. The system is used in clients who have highly variable respiratory patterns and are usually critically ill. Both high and low concentrations of oxygen can be administered with a high-flow system.

Venturi mask (Fig. 6-8)

Indications	Advantages/ Disadvantages	Nursing Considerations
Low oxygen concentrations need to be administered precisely	Delivery of exact Fio_2	Observe face for pressure sores
Clients with COPD	Humidification	Remove mask every 2-3 hours to clean face
	Does not dry oral/nasal mucosa	Multicolored adaptors provided with the mask indicate the liter flow required to deliver a prescribed O_2 level
	Mask must be fit snugly	
	May be hot or confining	
	Must be removed to eat	

Figure 6-8
Venturi mask
(From Wade JF: Comprehensive respiratory care, ed 3, St Louis, 1982, The CV Mosby Co.)

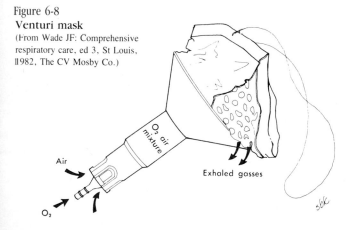

Air

O_2 air mixture

O_2

Exhaled gasses

Humidifiers
Cold bubble humidifier

Description	Nursing Considerations
Used with nasal cannulas, oxygen masks, nasal catheter	Do not use with tracheostomy
	Empty jar before refilling
Delivers 20%-40% humidity	Check water level every 8 hours

Cascade humidifier

Description	Nursing Considerations
Delivers 100% humidity	Monitor temperature control frequently
Temperature set at 37° C	
Used in mechanical ventilators	Check water level every 2 hours
	Empty cascade before refilling
	Drain excess water from tubing frequently

Room humidifier

Description	Nursing Consideration
Available in cool mist, centrifugal, vaporizer, or ultrasonic steam	Empty every 8 hours
Can be used with nasal cannula, oxygen masks	Do not add water to humidifier
Particle size ultrasonic: 3-10 μ centrifugal: >10 μ	Inspect for growth of mold and other organisms: colonization and nebulization of organisms are possible. Refer to specific infection control guidelines of the institution
	Humidity is not controlled
	For deposition to lower airways, 1-5 μ particle size is preferred (McPherson, 1981, p. 121)

Nebulizers
Pneumatic (jet) reservoir nebulizers

Description	Nursing Considerations
(Available heated and cool) Heated: 100% humidity Cool: 40%-50% humidity Safe for long-term use Can deliver variable O_2 concentrations: 35%-100%	The greater the volume of air entrained into the unit, the greater the water output (Harper, 1981, p. 235) Check water level every 2 hours
Available disposable and non-disposable	Drain large-bore tubing every 2 hours Empty jar before refilling

Ultrasonic nebulizers

Description	Nursing Considerations
Used for intermittent therapy for thick secretions Delivers 100% humidity Loosens secretions Density of mist and particle size allows penetration to the smaller distal airways	Client should not be left unattended during treatment Observe for signs of acute respiratory distress from airway obstruction Client may develop bronchospasm

References

Harper RW: A guide to respiratory care physiology and clinical applications, Philadelphia, 1981, JB Lippincott Co.

McPhersen SP: Respiratory therapy equipment, St Louis, 1990, The CV Mosby Co.

Bibliography

American Heart Association: Textbook of advanced cardiac life support, Dallas, 1987, The Association.

Perry AG: Oxygenation. In Perry AG and Potter PA, editors: Clinical nursing skills and techniques, St Louis, 1986, The CV Mosby Co.

Shapiro BA, Harrison RA, and Front CA: Clinical application of respiratory care, ed 3, Chicago, 1985, Yearbook Medical Publishers, Inc.

Spearman CB, Sheldon RL, and Egan DF: Egan's fundamentals of respiratory therapy, St Louis, 1982, The CV Mosby Co.

Springhouse Corporation: Clinical pocket manual respiratory care, 1985, Springhouse, Pennsylvania, Springhouse Corporation.

Springhouse Corporation: Respiratory care handbook, 1989, Springhouse, Pennsylvania, Springhouse Corporation.

Ventilation

Mechanical Ventilation

Use of mechanical ventilation is now an ordinary level of care for clients managed in the ICU and on general nursing care divisions. The client requiring mechanical ventilation presents a unique challenge for the clinician providing the care. The clinician should have a thorough knowledge of the mechanical ventilator, modes of mechanical ventilation, complications associated with mechanical ventilation, and nursing care considerations.

There are several indications for mechanical ventilation (Trulock and Schuster 1986).

Indication	Assessment Finding
Neuromuscular disease	Inspiratory pressure <25 cm H_2O
Guillian-Barré syndrome	Vital capacity <15 ml/kg
Myasthenia gravis	Respiratory rate >30-40/minute
Central airway obstruction	Presence of inspiratory stridor
Lung parenchymal or airway disease	Pao_2 <60 mm Hg, with Fio_2 >0.6
	$Paco_2$ >45 mm Hg; pH <7.3
ARDS, pneumonia, asthma pulmonary edema,	Respiratory rate >30-40/minute
Circulatory failure	As in parenchymal lung disease
Myocardial infarction	
Cardiogenic shock	
Acute exacerbations of COPD	Pao_2 <35-45 mm Hg despite O_2 therapy
	pH <7.2-7.25
	Respiratory rate >30-40/minute

Types of Mechanical Ventilation

Mechanical ventilators are divided into two major categories: negative pressure and positive pressure ventilators. Negative pressure ventilators are primarily used with clients who have neuromuscular disease and central nervous system disorders. Positive pressure ventilators include volume cycled, pressure cycled, timed cycled, and high-frequency ventilators.

NEGATIVE PRESSURE VENTILATORS

Definition	Types	Indications	Nursing Considerations
Negative pressure is applied intermittently or continuously to the thorax or entire body. Pressure changes between the external chest wall and ventilator cause inspiration	Iron lung Cuirass Poncho Bodywrap	Neuromuscular disease CNS disorders Spinal cord injuries/ fractures COPD	Client usually does not require artificial airway Client may develop decreased venous return, decreased cardiac output, and peripheral vascular collapse from negative pressure applied to abdominal cavity. Fio_2 can be added via nasal cannula or mask

POSITIVE PRESSURE VENTILATORS

Definition	Types	Indications	Nursing Considerations
Time cycled: Inspiration is delivered over a specific preset time	1.3 PB-Emerson BP 200	Used in neonates and children	Constant inspiratory phase Variable pressure and volume dependent on inspiratory cycle
Pressure cycled: Inspiration is delivered until a preset pressure has been reached	Bennett PR 2	Short-term ventilation	May result in pneumothorax in clients with decreased lung compliance Should not be used in clients with restrictive or bolus lung disease, since it may cause pneumothorax
Volume cycled: Inspiration is delivered until a preset tidal volume has been reached	MA1,MA2 MA 2+2 BEAR 2-5 PB 7200 Servo 900C	Acute respiratory failure COPD ARDS	Reliable tidal volume Responsive to changes in lung compliance

Definition	Types	Indications	Nursing Considerations
High frequency ventilator:	Bronchopleural fistula	See modes of ventilation: high frequency ventilation	
Delivers small tidal volumes at high respiratory rates	Upper airway reconstruction		
Includes high frequency jet ventilation; high-frequency positive pressure ventilation and high-frequency oscillation			

Nursing Care of the Client Receiving Mechanical Ventilation

Clients receiving mechanical ventilation are dependent on the nurse to maintain their airway and ventilator. The nurse must be familiar with the symbols and definitions of ventilator parameters (Table 7-1) and the multiple modes available for mechanical ventilation (Tables 7-2 and 7-3). Care measures should focus on airway maintenance, adequate oxygenation and carbon dioxide removal, comfort measures, relief of anxiety, assistance with communication, and client and family education (Tables 7-4 and 7-5). Some of the nursing diagnoses frequently associated with these clients are listed on p. 199. The box on p. 201 lists some complications associated with mechanical ventilation.

Text continued on p. 199.

Table 7-1 Ventilator parameters

Parameter	Definition	Ventilator Setting
Tidal volume (V_T)	Amount of air inspired and expired with each breath	10-15 cc/kg of body weight
Respiratory rate (R for RR)	Number of breaths delivered per minute	10-16 breaths per minute
Fraction of inspired oxygen (Fio_2)	Amount of oxygen the client receives	.21%-1.0% to maintain Pao_2 60-80 torr (Fernandez and Cherniak, p. 175)
Positive end expiratory pressure (PEEP)	Positive pressure applied at end expiration to improve oxygenation	+3-5 cm H_2O may be used to approximate physiologic PEEP* May require higher levels >5 cm H_2O in respiratory failure, e.g., ARDS
Sigh	Larger than normal breath to provide hyperinflation. Helps prevent atelectasis	Usual by twice the tidal volume breath About 10-15 ml/kg Rate is usually set at 10-15 times per hour (Dupuis, 1986)
Sensitivity	Determines the inspiratory effort required to trigger the ventilator	Set to respond to an inspired volume of less than 1% of the client's tidal volume (Dupuis, 1986)

*Some clinicians believe that the ETT with inflated cuff creates a closed system with the ventilator and does not require 3-5 cm of PEEP.   *Continued.*

Table 7-1 Ventilator parameters—cont'd

Parameter	Definition	Ventilator Setting
Peak airway pressure	The maximal pressure level required to deliver the desired tidal volume	<40 cm H_2O
I:E Ratio	Comparison of inspiratory to expiratory time	Normally set 1:1, 1:2, or 1:3 Example: inspiration 2 seconds, expiration 4 seconds: then I:E = 1:2 (Dupuis, 1986)
Exhaled minute ventilation $\dot{V}_E$	Measures the exhaled minute ventilations in liters	Alarm set at 15% greater than client's average $\dot{V}_E$

Table 7-2 Modes of mechanical ventilation

Mode	Definition	Indications	Comments
Control mode (CM)	Preset tidal volume and preset rate delivered to the client regardless of the client's respiratory effort. The client cannot initiate breaths or change the ventilatory pattern	Neuromuscular disease Drug overdose Reduction of work of breathing	Client may require sedation to reduce competition with the ventilator Rarely used
Assist control mode (A/C) Continuous mandatory ventilation (CMV)	Preset tidal volume and preset rate is delivered to the client. The client can initiate breaths that are delivered at the preset tidal volume	Reduction of work of breathing Respiratory muscle fatigue COPD Postanesthesia	Client may need sedation to reduce spontaneous breaths (Vasbinder-Dillon, 1988)

Continued.

Table 7-2   Modes of mechanical ventilation—cont'd

Mode	Definition	Indications	Comments
Intermittent mandatory ventilation (IMV)	Preset tidal volume and preset rate is delivered to the client. Between machine breaths the client can breath spontaneously at their own tidal volume	Primary ventilatory mode Used to wean clients from mechanical ventilation	Client should be assessed for synchrony with the mechanical ventilator. Monitor the client's inspiratory effort to synchronize with the ventilator's inspiratory cycle
Synchronized intermittent mandatory ventilation (SIMV)	The IMV mode is synchronized with the client's spontaneous breathing to reduce competition between machine-delivered and client-spontaneous breaths	Primary ventilatory mode Used to wean clients from mechanical ventilation	Client synchrony with the ventilator is improved

Pressure support ventilation (PSV)	Provides positive pressure during the inspiratory cycle of a spontaneous inspiratory effort (Weilitz, 1989)	Weaning clients with COPD	There is not a preset respiratory rate. The clinician must assess for muscle fatigue and potential periods of apnea. Improved client-ventilator interaction and client comfort.
High-frequency positive pressure ventilation (HFPPV)	Tidal volume of 2-5 cc/kg delivered through an insufflation catheter or pneumatic valve attached to the endotracheal tube at rate of 60-100 cycles/minute	Bronchopleural fistula During bronchoscopy, laryngoscopy Anesthesia during lithotripsy	Requires a special insufflation catheter or pneumatic valve attached to the ETT Clients may have increased amounts of tracheobronchial secretions

Continued.

Table 7-2 Modes of mechanical ventilation—cont'd.

Mode	Definition	Indications	Comments
High-frequency jet ventilation (HFJV)	Tidal volume of 3-7 cc/kg are delivered at rate of 60-600 times/minute as small jets of air (Weilitz, 1989)	Reconstructive upper airway surgery Bronchopleural fistula	Clients experience increased oral secretions Requires frequent assessment of sputum consistency and character Adequate cuff seal is important to prevent aspiration Requires close monitoring of cardiopulmonary status Auscultation of heart and lung sounds will be more difficult because of pulsing sound of ventilator
High-frequency oscillation (HFO)	Delivers tidal volume of 1-3 cc/kg at respiratory rates of 30-3000 cycles/minute	Respiratory distress syndrome Internal pulmonary physiotherapy	Monitor for increased secretions

Inverse ratio ventilation (IRV)	Increased inspiratory phase and shortened expiratory phase; I:E ratio of 2:1 or greater	Refractory hypoxemia ARDS Diffuse lung disease	Monitor secretions for character and consistency because of reduced humidification Clients have a feeling of fullness Clients usually require sedation to increase comfort and reduce anxiety Client may experience hypotension Closed suction system may be beneficial
Airway pressure release ventilation (APRV)	Variation of the IRV method Airway pressure is released intermittently to allow passive CO_2 elimination (Weilitz, 1989)	Acute lung injury	See IRV

Continued.

Table 7-2 Modes of mechanical ventilation—cont'd

Mode	Definition	Indications	Comments
Mandatory minute ventilation (MMV)	A constant minute ventilation ($\dot{V}_E$) is maintained as the ventilator monitors spontaneous tidal volume and respiratory rate and offers ventilatory support as needed to maintain the preset minute ventilation	Weaning	Monitor for respiratory rate Assess a/A ratio to determine minute ventilation needs
Independent lung ventilation (ILV)	Ventilation technique that ventilates each lung separately	Unilateral pathology Massive hemoptysis Thoracic trauma	Maintain correct positioning of double lumen tube Client requires a clinician at the bedside at all times Client may require restraints or sedation

Table 7-3 PEEP and CPAP

Mode	Definition	Indications	Comments
Positive end expiratory pressure (PEEP)	Positive pressure applied at end expiration	Improves oxygenation Improves distribution of ventilation Recruitment of alveoli Increases FRC	May cause decreased venous return and hypotension Monitor blood pressure, heart rate High levels of PEEP (>5 cm H_2O) may cause barotrauma Observe for pneumothorax
Continuous positive airway pressure (CPAP)	PEEP applied during spontaneous respiration	Improves oxygenation Improves distribution of ventilation Recruitment of alveoli Increases FRC	May cause hypotension Client may feel short of breath

Table 7-4 Ventilator alarms

Alarm	Definition	Potential Cause
High pressure	Pressure required to ventilate exceeds preset pressure	Pneumothorax Excessive secretions Kinked ventilator tubing Decreased lung compliance
Low pressure	Resistance to inspiratory flow is less than preset pressure	Client disconnected from ventilator Break in ventilator circuit
Low exhaled volume	Exhaled tidal volume drops below preset amount	Leak in system Increasing airway resistance Decreased lung compliance
Rate/Apnea	Respiratory rate drops below preset level Apneic period exceeds set time interval.	Client fatigue Decreased respiratory rate resulting from medication Change in level of consciousness
Fio_2	Indicates Fio_2 drift from preset range. Available on the Servo 900 C ventilator	Client disconnected from oxygen source Break in ventilator circuit

Table 7-5 Troubleshooting mechanical ventilation (Martz et al, 1984)

Ventilator Alarm	Possible Cause	Nursing Interventions
Sudden rise in peak airway pressure	Coughing	Clear secretions by suctioning
	Airway plugging	Reposition client
	Changes in client position	Assess breath sounds, chest wall movement
	Pneumothorax	Verify placement of endotracheal tube
	Incorrect endotracheal tube position	Assess breath sounds
		Verify cm level of endotracheal tube
	Kinked ventilator circuit	Check circuit; unkink tubing
	Excessive water in ventilator circuit	Drain tubing
Gradual increase in peak airway pressure	Decreasing lung compliance	Evaluate breath sounds; suction
	Exacerbation of acute process	Check for reversible causes: airway plugging, bronchospasm

Continued.

Table 7-5 Troubleshooting mechanical ventilation (Martz et al, 1984)—cont'd

Ventilator Alarm	Possible Cause	Nursing Interventions
Sudden decrease in peak airway pressure	Client disconnected from ventilator	Check for disconnection
	Leak in ventilator circuit	Evaluate circuit connections; tighten loose connections
Change in minute ventilation or tidal volume		
Decrease	Leak in endotracheal tube cuff	Check cuff seal
	Airway secretions	Suction excessive secretions
	System leak	Check circuit connections
	Increased respiratory rate	Evaluate respiratory rate
Increase	Hypoxia	Evaluate for signs of hypoxia. Evaluate need to obtain ABG sample or monitor pulse oximetry
Change in respiratory rate	Client anxiety	Reassure client
	Increased metabolic demand	Evaluate body temperature, heart rate, and rhythm
	Hypoxia	Obtain ABG or monitor pulse oximetry

Nursing Diagnosis	Nursing Considerations
Ineffective airway clearance related to excessive, thick secretions	Suction frequently
	Assess breath sounds to aid in determining need for suctioning
	Provide adequate hydration to prevent airway secretion plugging
	Assess secretions for consistency and character
	Monitor endotracheal tube for correct positioning noting cm level
	Secure ventilator circuit to client's gown to prevent pulling on artifical airway
	Maintain cuff pressure and seal at 18 mm Hg or less
Impaired gas exchange related to alveolar hypoventilation	Improve ventilation/ perfusion ratios by positioning client with good lung down.
	Encourage elevation of head of bed to 30-90 degrees as tolerated
	Encourage client to sit up in chair as tolerated, to increase ventilation

Nursing Diagnosis	Nursing Considerations
	Monitor oxygen saturation during nursing care and exercise; use pulse oximetry as available
Potential for infection related to artifical airway and mechanical ventilation	Provide sterile suctioning
	Never drain ventilator circuit water into humidifier jar
	Always drain excessive water in tubing before repositioning client
	Drain water away from client into appropriate receptacle
	Change suction canisters every 24 hours
	Provide endotracheal tube care and tracheostomy care as indicated
	Place waterproof field over client's chest or on the bed for ventilator circuit during suctioning
Alteration in nutrition related to artificial airway and interference with eating	Monitor total protein (>3.5 g/dl); serum albumin (>3g/dl); total lymphocyte count (>1200 cells/cm) (Selevanov et al., 1983)

Nursing Diagnosis	Nursing Considerations
	Monitor CO_2 production to determine carbohydrate load in feedings
	Weigh client daily
Alteration in communication related to artificial airway	Provide alternative means of communication, e.g., magic slate, pen and pad, and communication board
	Spend time with client and family to allow them to express needs

Complications Associated with Clients Receiving Mechanical Ventilation

Airway
  Tracheal necrosis
  Tracheal stenosis
Barotrauma
  Pneumothorax
  Pneumomediastinum
  Subcutaneous emphysema
Cardiovascular
  Hypotension
  Arrhythmias
  Decreased cardiac output
Gastrointestinal
  Aspiration
  GI bleeding
  Malnutrition
    Gastric distention
    Diarrhea
Infection
  Nosocomial infection
  Upper respiratory infection
Immobility
  Muscle wasting
  Deep vein thrombosis
  Pulmonary emboli
  Decubitus ulcers
Other
  Atelectasis
  Increased ADH production
  Fluid and electrolyte imbalance

Using a self-inflating resuscitation bag

"Bagging" is the technique of using a self-inflating resuscitation bag to ventilate the client manually (Fig. 7-1). A bag should be at the bedside of every client requiring mechanical ventilation or those at risk for respiratory failure. Bagging is used to hyperinflate and hyperoxygenate the client before suctioning, when ambulating the client on mechanical ventilatory support, and when the ventilator has mechanical failure. It is also used to assist the client who is asynchronous with the ventilator, who has dyspnea, or is disconnected from the ventilator for tubing changes or other procedures.

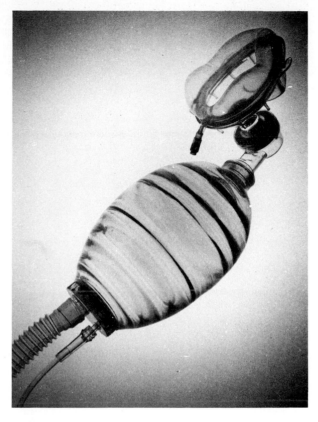

Figure 7-1
Bag valve mask.
(From Sheehy S: Manual of emergency care, ed 3, St Louis, 1990, The CV
Mosby Co). Photo by Richard Lazar.

During the procedure the clinician must observe the spontaneous respiratory effort and augment the tidal volume. As the client initiates a breath, the clinician compresses the bag fully. If the client's respiratory rate is too rapid to administer a deep breath, the clinician bags at a rate greater than the client's respiratory rate. This will allow the clinician to regain control of the respiratory rate and tidal volume (Fig. 7-2).

The self-inflating bags require 15 LPM flow to ensure rapid reinflation after delivery of a breath. The bag should be connected to its own flow meter and available at all times.

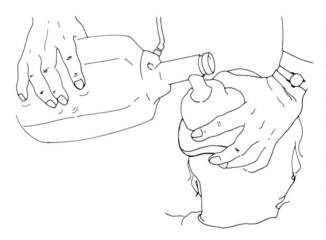

Figure 7-2
Ventilation bag in use.
(From Wade JF: Comprehensive respiratory care, ed 3, St Louis, 1982, The CV Mosby Co).

Single-bottle system

The single-bottle system (Fig. 7-3) acts as both the water sea
and the collection bottle. The bottle is partially filled with 30(
500 ml of sterile water, and the distal end of the glass tube
submerged 1 to 2 cm underwater. The proximal end of the glas
tube is connected to a latex tube approximately 6 feet in lengtl
As the client exhales, air in the thorax is forced out through th
chest tube into the bottle. The air either dissolves in the fluid
bubbles through the fluid, escaping through the vent port. As th
client inhales, the water seal prevents air from entering the pleu
ral space through the chest tube.

The amount of force needed to exhale increases as the amour
of fluid in the bottle increases with chest drainage. When this in
crease occurs, the bottle can be emptied or a two-bottle systen
can be used.

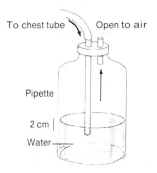

Figure 7-3
Single-bottle system.
(From Abels LF: Mosby's manual of critical care, St Louis, 1979, The CV Mos
Co).

Managing chest tubes

Clients receiving mechanical ventilation may require the insertion of a chest tube if a pneumothorax or tension pneumothorax develops. A chest tube can be inserted to remove air, blood, and fluid from the pleural space, allowing the collapsed lung to reexpand. Chest tubes are frequently inserted following thoracic surgery to drain the thorax and allow for lung reexpansion. The chest tube drainage system consists of a large-bore drainage tube, a collection bottle, and a water seal, which prevents air from entering and reaccumulating in the pleural space.

The position of the chest tube within the chest indicates what is to be drained. Chest tubes used to drain air are usually placed in the anterior chest at the midclavicular line in the second or third intercostal space. Chest tubes placed to drain fluid, blood, or effusions are lower in the chest at the midaxillary line in the fourth to sixth intercostal space. A No. 16 to No. 24 French tube is used to drain air, and a No. 28 to No. 36 French tube is used to drain liquids (Erickson, 1989).

Nursing responsibilities during the insertion of the chest tube include assisting the physician with the procedure and providing assurance and comfort for the client. The client and family should be educated about the procedure, the reason for the chest tube, the expected discomfort during the procedure, and the expected discomfort and limited mobility after the procedure. The client should be assured that he or she will be medicated, if possible, before the procedure and that comfort measures and positioning for pain relief will be carried out. The pleura is difficult to anesthetize; therefore, the client feels much pressure and discomfort during the chest tube insertion as the tube is advanced through the muscle and pleura.

After insertion, the chest tube is connected to a water-sealed drainage system. The chest tube is sutured in place, and an occulusive dressing of petrolatum gauze is applied.

The type of drainage system used (single-bottle, two-bottle, or three-bottle system) depends on the reason the chest tube is inserted. For a simple pneumothorax a single bottle system is sufficient. A two-bottle system is used when a large amount of draining is anticipated. The three-bottle system allows the addition of suction to aide in the removal of fluid or air.

Two-bottle system

A two-bottle drainage system is used when a large amount of drainage is anticipated. The first bottle is the collection bottle, the second bottle is the water seal. The tubes in the first bottle are short and do not extend into the fluid level. The second bottle is partially filled with 300-500 ml of sterile water, and the glass tube is submerged one to two centimeters below the fluid level as in the single bottle set-up. The bottles are set up in series to create the closed system (Fig. 7-4).

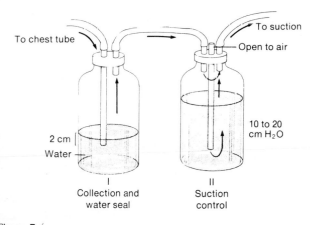

Figure 7-4
Two-bottle system.
(From Abels LF: Mosby's manual of critical care, St Louis, 1979, The CV Mosby Co).

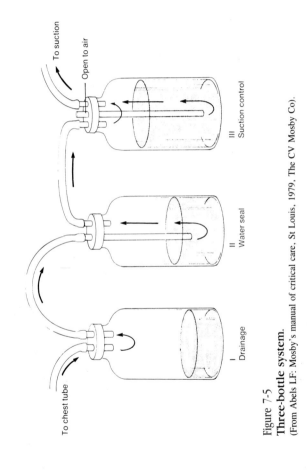

Figure 7-5
Three-bottle system.
(From Abels LF: Mosby's manual of critical care, St Louis, 1979, The CV Mosby Co).

Three-bottle system

A three-bottle system (Fig. 7-5) is set up when suction is needed, as in extensive pneumothorax or hemothorax. The third bottle is connected to the water seal bottle at the air vent and provides the suction control. The third bottle has a manometer submerged in the sterile water in the suction control bottle. The suction port is connected to a suction device.

When the suction is turned on, bubbling in the suction control bottle should occur. The depth of the underwater manometer is directly related to the suction on the client's pleura. The deeper the manometer, the more pressure exerted. The depth of the water in the suction control bottle (5 cm to 20 cm) determines the suction applied. Turning the suction device up higher will not increase the amount of suction; it will only increase the amount of bubbling in the suction control bottle. The amount of water in the suction control bottle should be monitored to ensure that the ordered amount of suction is maintained.

Disposable chest drainage systems

Plastic disposable chest drainage systems are available from many manufacturers. The disposable systems are single units with three chambers which can be used for one-, two-, and three-bottle systems. The first chamber corresponds to a single-bottle system; the first and second chambers are used if a two-bottle system is needed; and all three chambers are used if suction is indicated. Suction is added by connecting the air vent to a suction device (Fig. 7-6).

The client with a chest tube should be monitored for signs of respiratory distress, including the monitoring of respiratory rate, depth of respiration, and use of accessory muscles of respiration. The client may complain of chest pain and discomfort at the insertion site. Pain medication should be administered as ordered. The client should be encouraged to move and turn in the bed. Positioning the client in the Fowler's position will aid in the removal of air and fluid (Holloway, 1986).

The client with a chest tube should receive pulmonary hygiene. Frequent coughing and deep breathing help prevent atelectasis and pneumonia. The client may need to be premedicated before attempting these procedures.

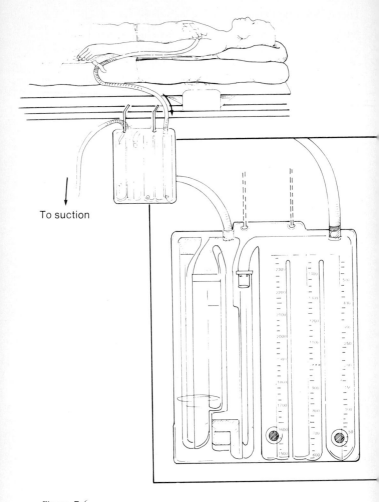

To suction

Figure 7-6
Pleur-evac.
(From Abels LF: Mosby's manual of critical care, St Louis, 1979, The CV Mosby Co).

The chest drainage system must be observed frequently to maintain patency. The collection chamber is observed for the amount, rate, and quality of drainage (Holloway, 1986). The level of the chest drainage should be monitored and marked on the drainage bottle hourly. If the drainage is greater that 100 ml per hour or frank bleeding is noted, the physician should be notified immediately.

The chest tube may also become clotted or obstructed. Draining the chest tube frequently, keeping the tube free of kinks, and keeping the tubing loosely coiled and flat in the bed will help prevent clotting and decreased chest drainage.

Table 7-6 includes other nursing care considerations and the nursing interventions for managing the chest drainage system.

Table 7-6   Troubleshooting the chest drainage system

Observation	Possible Cause	Nursing Interventions
Rise and fall of fluid in glass tube in water seal	Normal: rise on inhalation; fall on exhalation; on mechanical ventilation the normal fluctuations will be the opposite	Observe hourly to ensure chest tube drainage system is functioning properly Disconnect suction to determine rise and fall of fluid
Fluid column does not fluctuate	Lung is reexpanded Possible obstruction Kinked tubing or client lying on tubing	Check all connections Unkink tubing, milk/strip tubing if ordered; reposition client
Continuous bubbling	Leak in the system	Check all connections

	Increase in suction system setting	Check dressing; it should be occlusive Adjust suction system setting to achieve desired suction
Broken chest bottle		Do not clamp the chest tube unless the lung is nearly reexpanded. The end of the tube can be submerged in a cup of sterile water until another system is set up
Drainage stops	Obstruction or clot in the tubing	Gently milk the tubing to relieve the obstruction if ordered
Change in amount or color of drainage	Excessive bleeding	Notify the physician immediately Monitor blood pressure and pulse

Milking and stripping a chest tube

Milking and stripping a chest tube has become controversial since there is little evidence of its benefits (Holloway, 1986). Manually compressing the drainage tube and releasing it to help dislodge clots and obstructions can generate excessive pressures in the chest tube. Suction is transmitted back to the pleural space at levels high enough to actually cause tissue damage (Holloway, 1986). Stripping a chest tube involves lubricating about 12 inches of the tube with lotion, pinching the tube shut proximal to the chest, and while pinching the tube with the other hand, sliding it distally. The proximal hand is released while the distal occulusion is maintained, creating the suction. This sequence is repeated along the entire length of the tube. Milking the chest tube is gentle compression and massaging of the chest tube to dislodge and move drainage forward in the tube. In many institutions clinicians are allowed to milk a chest tube as needed; however, a physician's order is required for stripping a chest tube.

Chest tube removal

The chest tube is removed when the lung has reexpanded or the chest drainage has decreased significantly. The procedure should be explained to the client and family. Removal of a chest tube is usually painful. The client should be medicated about 30 minutes before the chest tube removal to maximize pain relief. The physician will perform the actual removal. The chest tube dressing and suture is removed. The client is instructed to take a deep breath and while Valsalva maneuver is performed, the tube is quickly removed and the site covered with a petroleum gauze dressing. An occulsive dressing is applied and can be changed 48-72 hours after the chest tube has been removed (Holloway, 1986).

Weaning from mechanical ventilation

Weaning from mechanical ventilation begins by assessing the client's ability to breathe without ventilatory support. Traditional weaning parameters (Table 7-7) assist the nurse in determining readiness. Client cooperation and effort are the key in establishing a baseline. The actual weaning process can be accompanied by T-piece trials, decreasing IMV rates or PSV weaning. Often a combination of techniques may be employed.

Nursing care during weaning requires constant observation by the nurse. The client needs reassurance and support. Preparing the client both psychologically and physiologically will increase the success of the weaning trials. The nurse must be alert for the assessment criteria that indicate when a weaning trial should be terminated.

Table 7-7   Weaning parameters

Parameter	Assessment Finding
Tidal volume (V_T)	4-5 cc/kg
Respiratory rate (R_f)	>12 and <30 breaths/minute
Minute ventilation ($\dot{V}_E$)	6-10 LPM
Negative inspiratory force (NIF)	>-20 cm H_2O
Forced vital capacity (FVC)	>15 cc/kg
Fraction of inspired oxygen (Fio_2)	<.50
Partial pressure of arterial oxygen (Pao_2)	>80 torr on Fio_2 <.50
Arterial oxygen saturation (Sao_2)	>90%
Maximum voluntary ventilation (MMV)	$>2 \times \dot{V}_E$
Positive end expiratory pressure (PEEP)	<5 cm H_2O

Clients should be rested before weaning trials begin. Do not attempt weaning during the night. Allow the client to have a normal sleep-wake pattern to reduce fatigue. Do not allow the client to become exhausted or overworked during the weaning trial. Elevate the head of the bed 30 to 90 degrees during the weaning trial. Do not wean in the supine position. Know the criteria for termination of weaning. Weaning methods are as follows:

Method	Technique	Nursing Considerations
T-piece trials	Alternating periods of spontaneous respiration with rest periods on the ventilator; usually alternating with assist control mode	Monitor baseline data
		Stay with client
		Monitor assessment parameters
	Start with 5-15 min trials 2-6 times/ day (Schuster, 1989)	Clients tolerating 1-2 hours of continuous T-piece trials usually can be extubated (Schuster, 1989)
	Small amounts of CPAP may be added to prevent airway closure and atelectasis	Assess breath sounds and secretions
		Monitor chest x-ray film for atelectasis
IMV	Gradual reduction of IMV rate as the client increases his or her own spontaneous breathing	Monitor for fatigue, decreased respiratory rate, and tidal volume
		Increased work of breathing is associated with breathing through high-resistance ventilator circuits.

Method	Technique	Nursing Considerations
		Monitor respiratory rate as indicator of increasing fatigue.
		Maintain RR <25 breaths per minute
PSV	Available on newer ventilators (e.g., PB 7200, Bear 5, Servo 900C)	Monitor for adequate respiratory rate and V_E. IMV backup rate may not be adequate to maintain $Paco_2$.
	Supports the inspiratory cycle of respiration with positive pressure decreasing work of breathing.	
	Positive pressure is usually set at 15-25 cm H_2O to maintain V_T of 10-15 ml/kg (Schuster, 1990).	
	If an IMV backup rate is used, it is decreased along with the PSV.	
	T-piece trials of 1-2 hours should be performed to evaluate client tolerance and ventilatory functions before extubation (Schuster, 1990)	

Assessment parameters and criteria for termination of weaning trials are as follows:

Client anxiety, discomfort, or decrease in level of consciousness

Blood pressure: increase in diastolic BP >100 mm Hg; fall in systolic BP of 20 mm Hg

Heart rate increase of >20 bpm

Respiratory rate increase of 10 breaths per minute

Tidal volume falls below 3-4 cc/kg

6 or more premature ventricular contractions (PVCs) per minute

ST segment changes

Pa_{CO_2} >55 torr

Pa_{O_2} <60 torr

pH <7.35

PCWP/LAP increase of >20 torr

Extubation procedure is as follows:

Begin early in the day

Explain procedure to client and family

Have client sit up in bed at 45-90 degree angle

Obtain baseline data: ABG, pulse, respiratory rate, blood pressure, cardiac rhythm, if monitored

Have equipment for reintubation at the bedside

Have a high humidity oxygen delivery system available at the bedside

Suction the airway and oropharynx

Be sure to suction any secretions that may have accumulated on the top of the cuff

Loosen endotracheal tube tape

Have the client take 2-3 deep breaths

Deflate the endotracheal tube cuff

Have client take a deep breath and cough as tube is removed

Provide high humidity oxygen source

Monitor client closely for stridor, laryngospasm, or need to reintubate

Encourage coughing and deep breathing

May sure a clinician skilled in intubation is available on the nursing unit for the first 1-2 hours after extubation

Intermittent positive pressure breathing

Intermittent positive pressure breathing (IPPB) is used to deliver medications, open distal alveoli, and help clear bronchial secretions. Clients using IPPB should be monitored for complications and adverse effects such as hypotension, tachypnea, dizziness, and tachycardia. The client should take slow deep breaths to prevent tachypnea. Monitor the client's heart rate, respiratory rate, and IPPB flow rates and pressures. Pneumothorax is a complication of excessive airway pressure. Decreased venous return, hypotension, and decreased cardiac output are common side effects of IPPB.

IPPB treatments have been used to reduce bronchospasms and prevent actelectasis in an effort to avoid intubation and mechanical ventilation. Treatments can vary from 10 to 30 minutes four to six times per day. The client should be observed during the treatment and provided with reassurance. The IPPB treatment makes many clients feel overinflated and uncomfortable.

Contraindications to IPPB include active tuberculosis, hemoptysis, postoperative thoracic surgery, increased intracranial pressure, pneumothorax, and subcutaneous emphysema. The absolute contraindication to IPPB is untreated tension pneumothorax.

Continuous positive airway pressure

Continuous positive airway pressure (CPAP) is maintenance of an airway pressure above atmospheric conditions during the inspiratory and expiratory cycle of a spontaneously breathing client (Becker, 1989). CPAP is used to improve oxygenation, increase FRC, and improve distribution of ventilation.

CPAP can be applied during T-piece weaning trials to help reduce atelectasis. It is also used at home to correct hypoxia and apnea associated with sleep apnea. Low levels of CPAP (5-15 cm H_2O) act as a pneumatic splint holding the oropharyngeal airway open (Mims, 1988). CPAP is applied using a tight-fitting nasal mask or nasal cannula. The procedure is usually tolerated well by the client.

References

Becker PJ: Oxygenation. In Perry AG and Potter PA, editors: Clinical nursing skills and techniques, ed 2, St Louis, 1989, The CV Mosby Co.

Dupuis YG: Ventilators: theory and clinical applications, St Louis, 1986, The CV Mosby Co.

Erickson RS: Mastering the ins and outs of chest drainage. I. Nursing 89, May, 37-43.

Fernandez E and Cherniack RM: The use and abuse of ventilators, Harrison's principles of internal medicine, Update II, 165-184, 1982.

Holloway NM: Nursing the critically ill adult, ed 2, Reading, Massachusetts, 1986. Addison-Wesley Publishing Co, Inc.

Martz KV, Joiner JW, and Shepherd RM: Management of the patient ventilator system: a team approach, ed 2, St Louis, 1984, The CV Mosby Co.

Mims BC: Advances in suctioning and airway care. The Ozark Chest Conference VIII, September 1988, Lewisville Texas.

Mims BC: You can manage chest tubes confidently, RN, January, 1985.

Selevanov V, Sheldon GF, and Fantini G: Nutrition's role in averting respiratory failure, J Respir Dis 4(9):29-32, 1983.

Schuster DP: Physiologic approach to initiating, maintaining, and weaning mechanical ventilatory support during acute respiratory failure, Am J Med 1989 88(3):268-278, 1990.

Trulock EP and Schuster DP: Acute respiratory failure. In Manual of Medical Therapeutics, ed 25, 1986, Boston, Little, Brown & Co.

Weilitz PB: New modes of mechanical ventilation, Critical Care Nursing Clinics 1(4):689-695, 1989.

Bibliography

Carroll PF: The ins and outs of chest drainage systems, Nursing 86, 16(12):26-33, December.

Spearman CB and Sheldon RL: Egan's fundamentals of respiratory therapy, ed 4, St Louis, 1982, The CV Mosby Co.

Stricter RM and Lynch JP: Complications in the ventilated patient, Clin Chest Med 9(1):127-139, 1988.

Swearingen PL, Sommers MS, and Miller K: Manual of critical care: applying nursing diagnosis to adult critical illness, St Louis, 1988, The CV Mosby Co.

Vasbinder-Dillon D: Understanding mechanical ventilators, Crit Care Nurse 8(7):42-56, 1988.

Why did that ventilator alarm go off? RN, July, 1985.

Winters C: Monitoring ventilator patients for complications, Nursing 88, June, 1988.

Pulmonary Rehabilitation

8

Pulmonary rehabilitation was defined in 1974 by the American College of Chest Physicians as "an art of medical practice wherein an individually tailored, multidisciplinary program is formulated which through accurate diagnosis, therapy, emotional support, and education, stabilizes or reverses both the physio and psychopathology of pulmonary diseases and attempts to return the patient to the highest possible functional capacity allowed by his pulmonary handicap and overall life situation." Each client is encouraged to reach his or her own level of success. A multidisciplinary approach is used including medicine, nursing, physical therapy, psychological counseling, education, and medication adjuncts.

The goals of pulmonary rehabilitation are (1) reduction of airflow obstruction, (2) prevention and treatment of complications, and (3) improvement in the quality of life. Clients are educated about their disease, how to manage acute exacerbations, and how to increase activities of daily living through regular exercise. The client's family or significant others should be included in the program to increase compliance and provide support.

Evaluation for a pulmonary rehabilitation program includes a diagnostic workup, evaluation of personal commitment, and assessment of resources. The diagnostic workup includes:

Diagnosis of symptomatic COPD

Complete pulmonary function studies

Chest radiograph

Electrocardiogram

Arterial blood bases—at rest and during exercise

Twelve- or 6-minute walk with oximetry

Cardiopulmonary or pulmonary stress test

Medical/surgical history

Sputum assessment

Serum theophylline level (if appropriate)

Educational Components

Pulmonary anatomy and physiology
Pathophysiology of COPD
Medication therapy
Bronchodilators
  Corticosteroids
  Antibiotics
  Metered dose inhalers
Smoking cessation
Oxygen therapy
Aerosol therapy
Energy conservation
Activities of daily living
Breathing exercises
Pulmonary hygiene
  Hydration
  Chest physiotherapy
    Postural drainage
    Vibration, cupping, rib shaking
Relaxation therapy
Nutritional counseling

The client is assessed for motivation and commitment to the program. Family support systems are evaluated for emotional support as well as commitment to the client's success. The client's ability to follow through on recommendations may be directly related to environmental and financial resources. If the client lives in an environment detrimental to his or her success (such as a family who continues to smoke), the client may be prevented from achieving success. Resources for medications, medical visits, the rehabilitation program, and oxygen therapy should be assessed. Social services are consulted to assist the client as needed.

The rehabilitation program teaches the client how to live with chronic lung disease in every aspect of his or her life. The multidisciplinary team approach provides the expertise to achieve this goal. The multidisciplinary team includes the physician, pulmonary clinical nurse specialist, physical therapist, psychologist, social worker, respiratory therapist, dietitian, occupational/activity therapist, client, and family/significant others. The team will assists the client in establishing long- and short-term goals, which helps the client define priorities. Success is measured as the client achieves and develops new goals.

Educational programs are comprehensive. A list of suggested topics are included in the box below. Education should be tailored to the individual client and family. Topics not currently part of the medical/nursing plan should be included. For example, even the client not receiving oxygen therapy should understand its use, safety precautions, and benefits. The more the client knows about his or her lung disease and its treatment, the more he or she may be able to participate actively in personal care.

Breathing Exercises

The goals of breathing exercises include decreased work of breathing, improved oxygenation, increased efficiency of breathing patterns and client control of breathing. Clients with respiratory disease must be taught how to relax and become conscious of their breathing patterns.

Diaphragmatic Breathing (Fig. 8-1)

The majority of the work of breathing (80%) is accomplished by the diaphragm (Modiak et al., 1975). This large, dome-shaped muscle becomes flattened and inefficient in clients with COPD. Teaching diaphragmatic breathing increases the client's awareness of the breathing pattern and improves efficiency. Instruct client as follows:

1. Lie in a supine or semi-Fowler's position
2. Place one hand on the middle of the stomach below the sternum
3. Place other hand on the upper chest
4. Inhale slowly through the nose. The stomach should expand. Note the movement with the hand over the stomach
5. Exhale slowly through pursed lips. The stomach should contract
6. Rest
7. Repeat

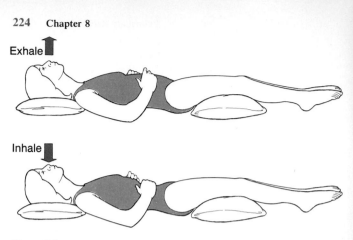

Figure 8-1
Diaphragmatic breathing.

The exercise should be repeated three to four times allowing for rest periods to prevent light-headedness from hyperventilating. Repeat the exercise four to six times a day until the skill is mastered, the client uses diaphragmatic breathing comfortably, and diaphragmatic breathing is the normal pattern of breathing.

Pursed Lip Breathing (Fig. 8-2)

Pursed lip breathing increases expiratory airway pressure, improves oxygenation, and helps prevent early airway closure. In addition, pursed lip breathing increases exhalation time, decreases respiratory rate, and allows the client to slow his or her breathing pattern. It is usually used in conjunction with diaphragmatic breathing. For pursed lip breathing, instruct the client as follows:

1. Assume a comfortable, relaxed position.
2. Inhale slowly through the nose. Keep the mouth closed.
3. Remember to use the diaphragmatic breathing technique.
4. Pucker the lips as if blowing out a candle, kissing, or whistling.
5. Exhale slowly, blowing through the pursed lips.
6. Exhalation should be at least twice as long as inhalation.
7. Rest.
8. Repeat.

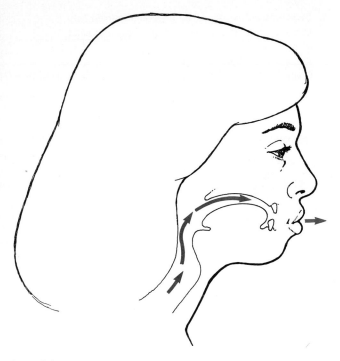

Figure 8-2
Pursed lip breathing.

Practice three to four breaths six to eight times a day until the technique is automatic. Pursed lip breathing is used during any exertional activity.

Chest Mobility Exercises

Chest mobility exercises help relax and loosen the accessory muscles of respiration. It is important to exhale on exertion during these exercises. Instruct client as follows.

Forward bending (Fig. 8-3)

1. Sit upright in a chair.
2. Inhale through the nose.
3. Raise arms above head.

4. Bend forward while exhaling through pursed lips.
5. Inhale as you sit up, raising arms above the head.
6. Rest.
7. Repeat six to eight times.

Caution: Do not bend over so far as to become dizzy or be uncomfortable.

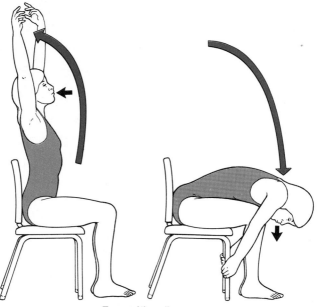

Forward bending

Figure 8-3
Forward bending.

Shoulder stretches

1. Sit upright in a chair.
2. Place hands behind your head with elbows to each side.
3. Inhale through the nose. Use diaphragmatic breathing technique.
4. Bend forward slowly while exhaling through pursed lips.
5. Bring elbows together.

6. Inhale through the nose as you slowly sit up stretching the elbows out to the original position.
7. Rest.
8. Repeat six to eight times.
   Caution: Do not bend over so far as to become dizzy or be uncomfortable.

Side bending (Fig. 8-4)

1. Sit upright in a chair.
2. Inhale slowly through the nose. Use diaphragmatic breathing technique.
3. Exhale slowly through pursed lips while bending trunk to the right. Arms are at sides.

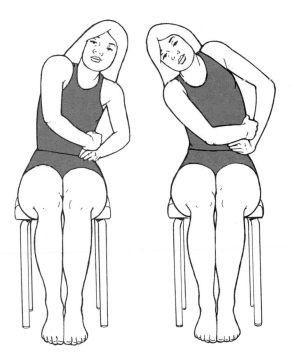

Figure 8-4
Side bending.

4. Inhale returning to upright position.
5. Repeat Steps *3* and *4*, bending to the left.
6. Rest.
7. Repeat entire sequence six to eight times.

Relaxing shoulder/neck muscles
Shoulder shrug (Fig. 8-5)

1. Sit in upright position.
2. Hang arms loosely at sides.
3. Inhale through the nose. Use diaphragmatic breathing techniques.
4. Exhale through pursed lips as you shrug your shoulders up toward your ears. Hold for 4 seconds.
5. Inhale as you relax your shoulders to the original position.
6. Rest for two to three normal breaths.
7. Repeat six to eight times.

Figure 8-5
Shoulder shrug.

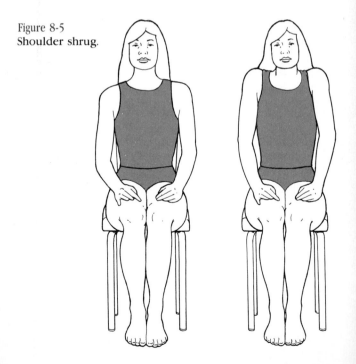

Head rotations

1. Bend head forward, with chin on chest.
2. Rotate head to right shoulder.
3. Rotate head backward.
4. Rotate head to left shoulder.
5. Return to beginning position.
6. Repeat six to eight times.
7. Rest.
8. Reverse starting to left first. Repeat entire exercise.
   This should be a slow continuous movement. Remember to breathe slowly while rotating the head.

Head turns (Fig. 8-6)

1. Sit in upright position.
2. Look straight ahead.
3. Rotate head to right looking toward the right underarm.
4. Return to forward position.
5. Rotate head to left looking toward the left underarm.
6. Return to forward position.
7. Rest.
8. Repeat eight to ten times.
   Remember to keep breathing slowly while repeating the exercise.

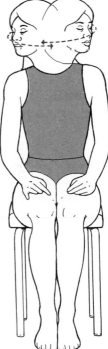

Figure 8-6
Head turns.

Strengthening Exercises for the Diaphragm and Abdomen
Leg lifts (Fig. 8-7)

1. Lie flat on back using a pad or mat on a hard surface such as the floor.
2. Bend right knee. Place foot flat on the floor.
3. Extend left leg straight.
4. Lift leg slowly. Exhale slowly through pursed lips. Bend knee slightly if uncomfortable.
5. Return leg to floor.
6. Bend left leg. Place foot flat on floor.
7. Extend right leg.
8. Lift leg slowly, exhaling through pursed lips. Bend knee slightly if more comfortable.
9. Return leg to the floor.
10. Caution: Keep back flat on the floor. Only lift one leg at a time, keeping the other knee bent with the foot flat on the floor.
11. Repeat five times for each leg.
12. Gradually increase repetions to 25 lifts for each leg.

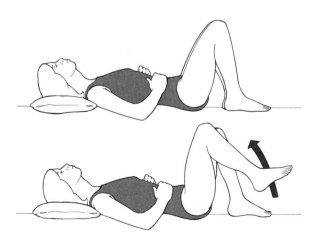

Figure 8-7
Leg lifts.

Knee-chest (Fig. 8-8)

1. Lie flat on back using a mat or pad on a hard surface, such as the floor.
2. Bend both knees keeping feet flat on the floor.
3. Inhale through the nose.
4. Exhale through pursed lips while bringing knees up to the chest.
5. Clasp hands around knees pulling gently toward chest.
6. Inhale while lowering feet to floor. Keep knees bent.
7. Rest.
8. Repeat four to six times.
9. Gradually increase until 15-20 exercises can be accomplished.

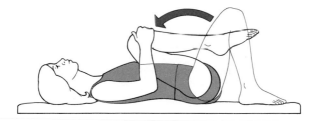

Figure 8-8
Knee-chest.

Sit-ups/crunches (Fig. 8-9)

1. Lie flat on back using a mat or pad on a hard surface such as the floor.
2. Bend both knees, keeping feet flat on the floor.
3. Place arms across chest or hands behind head.
4. Exhale through pursed lips while you sit up, slowly crunching shoulders forward.
5. Keep the small of the back on the floor.
6. Lower yourself back to the floor.
7. Inhale through the nose.
8. Repeat slowly and continuously. Start with four to six repetitions building to 20-25.

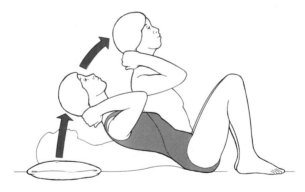

Figure 8-9
Sit-ups/crunches.

Inspiratory Muscle Training (Fig. 8-10)

Clients with COPD have limited strength and endurance of their inspiratory muscles. Specific training targeted at the inspiratory muscle can be beneficial in improving respiratory muscle function, reducing respiratory muscle fatigue and improving exercise tolerance. This is accomplished through the use of inspiratory muscle training devices such as the Pflex™ or Threshold™ models.

The clients are instructed to use the devices for 5 to 20 minutes daily. By progressively breathing through a variable orifice (Pflex) or a constant inspiratory pressure load (Threshold), an increased workload is placed specifically on the inspiratory muscles. Clients should be cautioned not to overbreathe, since overbreathing causes respiratory alkalosis.

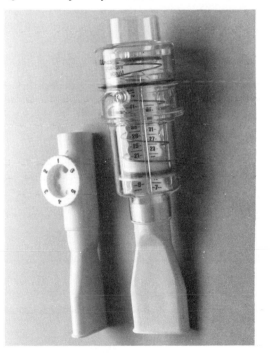

Figure 8-10
Inspiratory muscle training devices. *Left,* Pflex; *Right,* threshold.

Although the client's exercise capacity may be increased, additional research is needed to address the benefit of inspiratory muscle trainers in a pulmonary rehabilitation program.

Establishing an Exercise Program

The exercise program is determined by the pulmonary rehabilitation medical director based on the evaluation data. The prescription for each client should include the intensity of the exercise, the duration of a single exercise session, the frequency of the exercise sessions, e.g., number of times per week, and the mode of exercise. Frequently prescribed exercises include stationary bicycling, walking either on a track or treadmill, and using an arm ergometer.

The client usually performs a combination of these exercises, including warm-up and cool-down periods and stretching exercises. The goal for the client is 20 to 30 minutes of continuous exercise at 70% to 85% of the age-predicted maximal heart rate (see box). Some clients will be symptom-limited as determined by their exercise stress test. Continuous oximetry is used to monitor saturation levels, which are maintained at greater than 85%-90%.

Calculating Age-Predicted Maximal Heart Rate

(220 − Age) × Desired Percentage
Example: 50-year old client
        Plan to exercise at the 80th percentile
        220 − 50 = 170
        170 × .80 = 136
        Target heart rate: 136
Maximal heart rate for a 50-year-old client at the 80th percentile = 136

References

American Thoracic Society: Pulmonary rehabilitation: Official ATS statement, Am Rev Respir Dis 124:663, 1981.

Modiak M et al: Better living and breathing: a manual for patients, St Louis, 1975, The CV Mosby Co.

Bibliography

Belman MJ: Exercise in chronic obstructive lung disease, Clin Chest Med 7(4):583-593, 1986.

Clanton TL et al: Inspiratory muscle conditioning using a threshold loading device, Chest 87:62-66, 1985.

Glover DW and Glover MM: Respiratory therapy: basics for nursing and the allied health professions, St Louis, 1978, The CV Mosby Co.

Hodgkin JE, Zoin EG, and Conners GL: Pulmonary rehabilitation guidelines to success, Boston, 1984, Butterworth Publishers.

Larson JL et al: Inspiratory muscle training with a threshold breathing device in patients with chronic obstructive pulmonary disease, Am Rev Respir Dis 318:689-696, 1988.

Larsen JL: Respiratory training with threshold, University of Illinois at Chicago, 1988, Cedar Grove, New Jersey, Health Scan Products.

Make BJ: Pulmonary rehabilitation: myth or reality? Clin Chest Med 7(4):1986.

Petty TL: Intensive and rehabilitative respiratory care, Philadelphia, 1974, Lea & Febiger.

Petty TL: Pulmonary rehabiliation—better living with new techniques, Respir Care 30(2):98-107, 1985.

Spearman CB and Sheldon RL: Chronic care and rehabiliation of respiratory failure. In Egan's fundamentals of respiratory therapy, ed 4, St Louis, 1982, The CV Mosby Co.

Respiratory Home Care

9

The current practice of returning clients to their homes sooner and the increase in technology that can be provided in the home present a challenge for the clinician faced with the task of discharge planning. Practices such as intravenous medication administration, hyperalimentation and mechanical ventilation, once thought to be available only in the hospital setting, are now seen more frequently in the home setting. Translating hospital procedures and practices into the home care setting can be frustrating and challenging to the hospital-based clinician. Many practices are modified in the home care setting. The modifications and recommendations for discharge planning for clients with respiratory care needs are presented in this chapter.

Benefits of Home Health Care

Allowing a client to return home promotes a sense of well-being and improves the client's self-esteem (Meany-Handy, and Loreau, 1984, p. 311). Most clients are less fearful in their homes, generally happier, and feel more in control of their own lives. The use of home health care has been shown to reduce the frequency of hospital admissions and, when compared to the cost of acute care, demonstrates a decline in resource consumption (Meany-Handy, and Loreau, 1984, p. 311).

Discharge Planning

The discharge planning process should begin as soon as the client is admitted to the hospital. The first step is to identify the reason the client was admitted and includes not only the medical diagnosis, but also the nursing diagnosis and any social or financial reasons. A client with asthma may have an acute excerabation because of lack of money to pay for the medication, or a client may return to the hospital because the family support system has broken down and no one is available to assist with the care. These are issues that frequently cannot be resolved in a short time period and need to be addressed within the first days of admission.

The discharge planning team for the respiratory client should include the client and family or support person, the nurse, pulmonary clinical nurse specialist, physician, respiratory therapist, physical and occupational therapist, social worker, speech therapist, home health care nurse, and durable medical equipment (DME) company.

Assessing the Client and Family for Home Care Needs

Preparing the client for home care requires careful evaluation of the nursing care and health maintenance needs. The client should be evaluated for his or her ability to provide daily hygiene, toileting, and nutritional needs. It is important to observe how the client handles these tasks in the hospital to determine what level of care or assistance will be needed in the home. Mobility needs are assessed and referred to the physical therapist for recommendations and discharge planning.

When it is determined that a client will be going home with a tracheostomy or requiring suctioning, for example, the client and family are then educated about the care required. Allowing the client or family to provide the care in the hospital setting will increase their understanding of the procedures, improve their skills, and decrease the chance of rehospitalization related to the specific procedure. It is important for the clinician to keep in mind the discharge plan and allow the client and family to perform the required tasks. Many times it will be easier for the clinician to do the procedure; however, the goal of returning the client to home as independent in daily living as possible must be the focus. If a skill cannot be mastered in the hospital setting, followup by the home health nurse or respiratory therapist will be essential in determining success.

When possible, home care equipment should be brought into the hospital for demonstration and operational instructions to the client and family. Equipment that cannot be brought into the hospital, such as a liquid oxygen system or a hospital bed, should be demonstrated to the family in the home setting by a qualified individual. Many DME and home health companies have client education materials, which they use to instruct the client and family.

In addition to assessing the ability of the client and family to learn and follow-through on nursing care procedures, the clinician should also assess the family as a unit. The age, health status, and work obligations of family members as well as other family commitments, should be taken into consideration. It would be unwise to send home a client who requires frequent nursing interventions if no one is available to provide care during the day. The social worker and clinician work together to assist the family in planning a workable, safe, and realistic plan for discharge.

The home environment is also assessed for running water, electricity, and adequate plumbing, heating, and cooling. The home's floor plan, size of doorways, and presense of stairs both into and inside the home are considered. Clients with COPD may not be able to climb the stairs required to reach their bedroom or ambulate the needed distance from the bedroom to the bathroom. Many times rearranging rooms is necessary; a client may have to be moved from an upstairs bedroom to the first floor or to a room closer to the bathroom. The size of the doorways and the physical arrangement of the furniture and hallways are important determinations if equipment such as wheelchairs, walkers, or hospital beds are needed. Carpeting may be a problem for clients with walkers and wheelchairs and those with portable oxygen cylinders. When many pieces of electrical equipment are anticipated, as with a client receiving mechanical ventilation, the number and type of electrical outlets need to be assessed to ensure that the equipment can be operated adequately and safely.

Careful planning and coordination of discharge needs provides the client with a safe and successful return to home. The success of the home care plan is many times reflected in the frequency of hospital readmissions.

Home Oxygen Systems

Oxygen systems available for home use include cylinders, liquid oxygen systems, and oxygen concentrators (Table 9-1). The type of system used should be determined based on the client's ability to use and understand the equipment as well as his or her activity level and oxygen liter flow (Table 9-2). Medicare clients are required to meet specific requirements to qualify for reimbursement of the costs of home oxygen (see box).

Table 9-1 Home oxygen systems

System	Advantages	Disadvantages
Liquid Oxygen System (Fig. 9-1)		Oxygen evaporation
	Portable	Costly when used at high flows or for increased
	Accurate	length of time
	Easy to read	May be difficult for client to refill portable unit
		from base unit

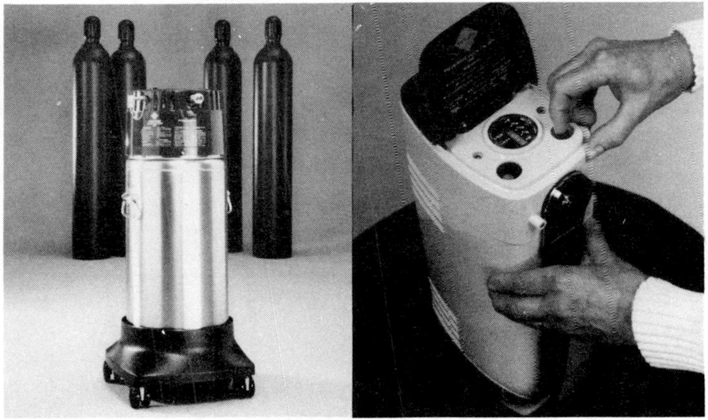

Figure 9-1
Liquid oxygen system.
(From Perry A and Potter P: Clinical nursing skills and techniques, ed 2, St Louis, 1990, The CV Mosby Co.)

Continued.

Table 9-1   Home oxygen systems—cont'd

System	Advantages	Disadvantages
Oxygen Cylinders	Least expensive delivery system if O_2 is needed 12 hours or less per day	Tanks are cumbersome; need to be changed frequently Limited portability
Oxygen Concentrators (Fig. 9-2)	High oxygen concentration Low noise level (quiet) Set monthly cost regardless of usage Low energy consumption	No portability Fio_2 above 3 L/min, Fio_2 can be less than 100%

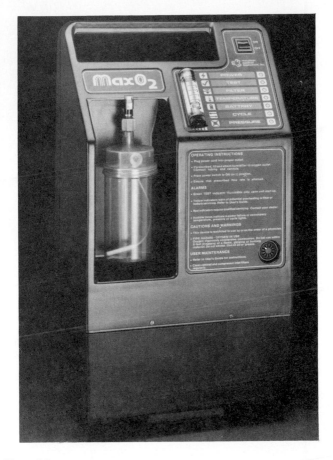

Figure 9-2
Oxygen concentrator.
(From Perry A and Potter P: Clinical nursing skills and techniques, ed 2, St Louis, 1990, The CV Mosby Co.) Courtesy Mountain Medical Equipment, Inc., Littleton, Co.

Table 9-2 Nursing care plan: client education: home oxygen therapy

Nursing Diagnosis	Expected Outcomes	Nursing Interventions
Knowledge deficit (ot home oxygen therapy) related to lack of exposure	Client will be able to state indication for home oxygen	Explain how oxygen gets into the blood. Explain client's specific alteration. Tell client his or her Pao_2 or Sao_2 with/without oxygen therapy.
	Client will be able to verbalize oxygen liter flow	Teach client prescribed liter flow.
	Client will be able to verbalize oxygen safety rules	Teach client oxygen safety rules. (See Chapter 6, p 127). Provide client with written rules
	Client will be able to demonstrate how to turn oxygen tank on and off, read oxygen pressure gauge, fill portable oxygen tank if liquid oxygen system is being used	Teach client how to use oxygen system at home. (May be done by home health nurse.) Make sure client is familiar with portable tank that will be used during transportion home. Provide written instructions
	Client will be able to verbalize time available for oxygen tank use based on liter flow	Teach client how to use tables in Appendix D. Provide written material for specific system used.

Medicare Qualifications for Home Oxygen

Pao_2 ≤55 mm Hg
   or
Sao_2 ≤85%
   or
Pao_2 =56 − 59 mm Hg
   and
Dependent edema suggesting congestive heart failure
   or
Cor pulmonale as evidenced on ECG or erythrocytosis as evidenced by hematocrit > 56%

Nocturnal Oxygen Therapy

Pao_2 ≤55 mm Hg during sleep
   or
Pao_2 falls greater than 10 mm Hg during sleep
   or
Sao_2 ≤85% during sleep or falls more than 5% during sleep

Exercise Oxygen Therapy

Pao_2 ≤55 mm Hg during exercise
   or
Sao_2 ≤85% during exercise

Durable medical equipment companies who accept Medicare assignments agree to accept the fixed cost established for home oxygen regardless of the system used. The DME company will provide the client with the most cost-effective system, which may not always be the preferred system to meet the client's needs. A prescription for oxygen therapy must include the respiratory diagnosis, type of system desired, flow rate, and frequency and duration of the oxygen therapy.

Example: Mary Jones
       Emphysema
       Liquid oxygen system with portable unit.
       2 L/min, 24 hr/day for 12 months

The physician should update the prescription for duration frequently. Medicare will not accept a prescription for lifetime. Selecting the type of system to be used should include consideration of client mobility, oxygen requirements, and duration of use.

Airway Care in the Home
Suctioning

Clients who require suctioning in the home modify the procedure from sterile to medically aseptic. The client may not use gloves during the procedure. Since the catheter is frequently used for multiple passes, it should be rinsed thoroughly with clean tap water. After rinsing the catheter, it is stored in a clean, self-sealing plastic bag. The same catheter may be used for the entire day. Catheters can be cleaned with hydrogen peroxide and water and used for multiple days. The procedure for cleaning suction catheters is as follows:

Rinse thoroughly in running water
Soak for 5 minutes in half strength hydrogen peroxide
Rinse thoroughly
Place in boiling water for 10-15 minutes
Remove from water and place on clean dry towel
Allow to air dry in a clean area
After completely dry, place in new plastic bag

Catheters with secretions that cannot be completely removed must be discarded. The client must be taught to carefully inspect the suction catheters for cleanliness.

Not all clients are able to use the clean technique when suctioning at home. Clients who are immunosuppressed, have an active infection, live in nonhygenic conditions, or are prone to frequent respiratory tract infections are not candidates for clean suction techniques. The nurse coordinating the discharge plan should carefully assess the client and family's ability to use clean techniques.

Tracheostomy Care

The major difference between home and hospital tracheostomy care is the use of clean technique. The actual procedure is identical. The client at home cleanses around the stoma with soap and water, usually as part of the normal hygiene routine. The inner cannula is cleansed with a mild soap and water and rinsed thoroughly with running tap water. Tracheostomy ties are changed when they become wet or soiled. The assistance of another person may be required. The guidelines for determining the type of technique a client should use are the same as those outlined in the section on suctioning.

Home Chest Physiotherapy

Home chest physiotherapy can be taught to a client's family member or friend preferably while the client is hospitalized, allowing the care provider time to develop the skill. If the care provider is unable to cup his or her hands appropriately, palm cups can be provided. Palm cups are soft, circular cups held in one's hands to provide the cupping. The techniques of chest physiotherapy are described in Chapter 4, Airway Management.

Postural drainage is accomplished by placing multiple pillows under the hips until the desired position is achieved. Some clients prefer a slant board or wedge-shaped pieces of foam. The slant board can be free standing or used against the bed. The physician will prescribe the appropriate position for drainage. See the discussion of chest physiotherapy in Chapter 4, Airway Management for a description of the postural drainage positions.

Percussion can also be accomplished by using an electrical percussor which has variable speeds for multiple intensity of percussion. Perscussion is applied to the prescribed area during the expiration phase of respiration. Continuous application during inspiration and expiration has little or no therapeutic effect.

Home Mechanical Ventilation

The client requiring long-term mechanical ventilation can be adequately cared for in the home. Careful assessment of the client, family, home environment and financial resources must be completed. Clients considered for home mechanical ventilation include those with neuromuscular disease and severe stable chronic obstructive pulmonary disease. Careful selection of the client is critical to the success of providing care in the home.

The criteria for client selection are as follows:

Stable health status (no plan for major therapeutic intervention within 30 days)

Pao_2 >60 mm Hg or Fio_2 ≤ .40

Stable arterial blood gases

Active cough/gag reflex

Tracheostomy tube in place for positive pressure ventilation

Requires infrequent suctioning

Free of infection

Client desires home ventilator care

Adequate family support

Adequate care providers

Adequate financial/insurance resources

The caregivers must be instructed in all aspects of providing care for the ventilator-dependent client. The box on the opposite page below lists the respiratory topics that must be mastered before discharge. In addition, the caregiver must learn how to provide nutritional needs, position and move the client, provide pressure relief measures, and assist with toileting needs. The commitment of the care providers and client are essential to a successful discharge.

The caregivers must be able to articulate and demonstrate all the skills necessary to provide home care before discharge. A multidisciplinary team of practitioners in medicine, nursing, respiratory therapy, physical therapy, and nutrition is essential to the success of the discharge. Not all ventilator-dependent clients are candidates for discharge to the home setting.

Knowledge that is Prerequisite to Preparation for Home Mechanical Ventilation

Respiratory Medication

Knowledge of actions
Side effects
Administration schedule
Administration method

Home Ventilator

Assembly and disassembly of the ventilator circuit
Cleaning the ventilator circuit
Ventilator settings
Control knobs
Alarm systems
What alarms indicate
Troubleshooting the ventilator

Oxygen Equipment

Type of equipment used
Oxygen safety
Use of manual resuscitating bag

Airway Care

Tracheostomy tube care
   Cuff care
   Changing a tracheostomy tube
Suctioning
   Tracheal suctioning
   Using a home suction machine
   Cleaning suction catheters

Chest Physiotherapy

   Using a chest percussor

Signs and Symptoms of Respiratory Infections

When to Call the Physician

Exercises

Chest mobility exercises
Range-of-motion exercises

Home Care Ventilators (Fig. 9-3)

Home care ventilators are designed to be portable and easy to use. They are small, usually 12 inches by 12 inches by 12 inches and weigh less than 40 pounds (Kacmarek, 1986). The ventilator operates from an A/C current, an internal D/C battery, or an external D/C battery. The knobs used to set the ventilator parameters are easy to use and read. The major disadvantages of home ventilators are the following: (1) they are limited in the flow rates and minute ventilations they can provide, usually less than 10 L/minute, (2) maintaining an accurate Fio_2 may be difficult, and (3) Fio_2 levels are limited to 40% or less. Despite these disadvantages, the ventilators are very effective in providing adequate ventilation and portability to a population of clients otherwise bound to hospital or institutional care.

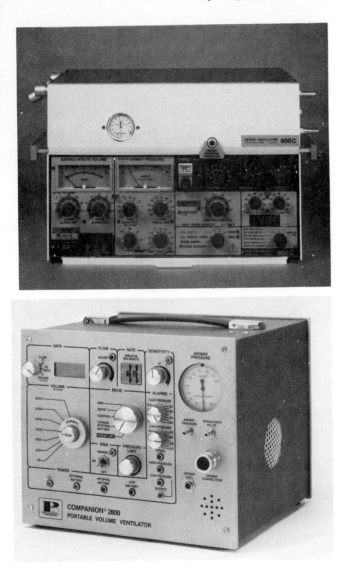

Figure 9-3
Home mechanical ventilators.

References

Kacmarek RM and Spearman CB: Equipment used for ventilatory support in the home, Respir Care 31(4):311-328, 1986.

Meany-Handy J and Loreau SL: The role of home care. In Hodgkin et al, editors: Pulmonary rehabilitation, Boston, 1984, Butterworth Publishers.

Bibliography

American Lung Association: Standards for the care of patients with chronic respiratory disease, New York, 1971, The Association.

American Thoracic Society: Standards for nursing care of patients with COPD, ATS News, Summer 1981:31.

Openbrier DR, Fuoss C, and Neil CC: What patients on home oxygen therapy want to know, Am J Nurs 2:198, 1988.

Openbrier DR, Hoffman LA, and Wesmiller SW: Home oxygen therapy, evaluation and prescription, Am J Nurs 2:198, 1988.

Perry AG and Potter PA: Clinical nursing skills and techniques, ed. 2 St Louis, 1990, The CV Mosby Co.

Prentice WS, Wilms D, and Harrison LB: Outpatient management of ventilator-dependent patients. In Hodgkin et al, editors: Pulmonary rehabilitation, Boston, 1984, Butterworth Publishers.

Santzker DR and Pingleton SK: Standards for the diagnosis and care of patients with chronic obstructive pulmonary disease (COPD) and asthma, Am Rev Res Dis 136(1):1987.

Gas Symbols

A	alveolar gas
B	barometric pressure
D	dead space
E	expired gas
F	fractional concentration of
f	frequency
I	inspired gas
R	respiratory quotient
STPD	standard conditions: temperature 0°C, pressure 760 mm Hg and water vapor 0
T	tidal gas
V	volume of gas

Blood Symbols

a	arterial
C	concentration of gas in blood
c	capillary
p	pulse oximetry
S	saturation of blood
v	venous
$\overline{v}$	mixed venous

Oxygenation/Ventilation Measurements

Note: Capital letters indicate the physical quantities, whereas the secondary symbol indicates the location.

A slash (-) over a symbol denotes mixed or mean value

A dot (.) over a symbol indicates a unit of time

a/A	arterial alveolar ratio
Ca_{O_2}	oxygen content of arterial blood
Cv_{O_2}	oxygen content of mixed venous blood
$C(a-v)_{O_2}$	arterial-venous oxygen content difference
Fi_{O_2}	fractional inspired oxygen concentration
P_B	barometric pressure
P_{H_2O}	water vapor pressure
P_{IO_2}	inspired oxygen partial pressure
P_{AO_2}	alveolar oxygen partial pressure
P_{CO_2}	alveolar carbon dioxide partial pressure
Pa_{O_2}	arterial oxygen partial pressure
Pa_{CO_2}	arterial carbon dioxide partial pressure
$P(A-a)_{O_2}$ or	
$A-aD_{O_2}$	alveolar arterial oxygen gradient
$P\bar{v}_{O_2}$	mixed venous oxygen partial pressure
$\dot{Q}$	cardiac output
$\dot{Q}s/\dot{Q}t$	percent shunt
Sa_{O_2}	arterial oxygen saturation
$S\bar{v}_{O_2}$	mixed venous oxygen saturation
$S\bar{p}_{O_2}$	pulse oximetry arterial oxygen saturation
$\dot{V}_E$	minute ventilation
$\dot{V}$	minute ventilation
V_D	physiologic dead space
V_D/V_T	dead space to tidal volume ratio
V_T	tidal volume
$\dot{V}/\dot{Q}$	ventilation/perfusion ratio
$\dot{V}_{CO_2}$	minute carbon dioxide production
$\dot{V}_{O_2}$	minute oxygen production
$\dot{V}_{CO_2}/\dot{V}_{O_2}$	respiratory exchange ratio

Appendix B   Formulas for Oxygenation/Ventilation Assessment

Oxygenation Assessment

A. Partial pressure of arterial oxygen (Pa_{O_2})
   1. Normal 80-100 torr
   2. Pa_{O_2} falls with age
      109 -.43 (age)
B. Oxygen carrying capacity
   Hgb $\times$ 1.34
C. Oxygen content
   Hgb $\times$ 1.34 $\times$ Sa_{O_2} + 0.003 $\times$ Pa_{O_2}
D. Arterial-venous oxygen content difference
   $C(a-\bar{v})O_2$

   1. $Ca_{O_2} = \dfrac{(Hgb \times 1.34 \times Sa_{O_2})}{100} + (Pa_{O_2} \times .003)$

   2. $C\bar{v}_{O_2} = \dfrac{(Hgb \times 1.34 \times Sa_{O_2})}{100} + (Pa_{O_2} \times .003)$

   If mixed venous gases are unavailable, assume 3.5-5.0
   vol % difference.
E. A-a gradient
   Alveolar air equation:

   $$P_{A_{O_2}} = (P_B - P_{H_2O}) \times Fi_{O_2} - \dfrac{Pa_{CO_2}}{.8 \ (RQ)}$$

   P_B — Barometric pressure (760)
   P_{H_2O} — Water vapor pressure (47)
   RQ — Respiratory quotient (.8)
   A-a gradient: $P_{A_{O_2}} - Pa_{O_2}$
   on room air = 10 mm Hg
   on Fi_{O_2} = 100 mm Hg
F. Shunt

   Classical: $Qs/Qt = \dfrac{Cc_{O_2} - Ca_{O_2}}{Cc_{O_2} - C\bar{v}_{O_2}}$

   Clinical: $Qs/Qt = \dfrac{(P_{A_{O_2}} - Pa_{O_2}) \ (0.003)}{(Ca_{O_2} - C\bar{v}_{O_2}) + (P_{A_{O_2}} \ Pa_{O_2}) \ (0.003)}$

Ventilation Assessment

A. Partial pressure of arterial carbon dioxide
   Pa_{CO_2} 35 − 45 torr

B. Minute ventilation ($\dot{V}_E$)
   $Rf \times V_T = \dot{V}_E$
   4-6 1/min normally

C. V_D/V_T

$$V_D/V_T = \frac{Pa_{CO_2} - P\overline{E}_{CO_2}}{Pa_{CO_2}}$$

D. Effective dynamic compliance

$$EDC = \frac{V_T}{PAP}$$

   Normal: Females: 35-45 ml/cmH$_2$O
             Males: 40-50 ml/cm H$_2$O

Appendix C   Oxyhemoglobin Dissociation Curve

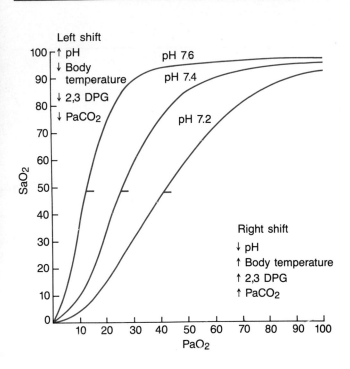

Appendix D   Oxygen Cylinder Time Tables*

E Cylinder

| | LPM | \multicolumn{5}{c}{Time in Hours} |
		1	2	3	4	5
Pressure Gauge Reading	2300 psi	10	5	3.5	2.5	2
	1800 psi	8.5	4.25	2.75	2.0	1.5
	1600 psi	7.5	3.75	2.5	1.5	1.25
	1200 psi	5.5	2.75	1.75	1.5	1.0
	1000 psi	4.5	2.25	1.5	1.0	54 min
	600 psi	2.75	1.5	50 min	40 min	30 min
	500 psi	2.5	1.25	45 min	30 min	15 min

H Cylinder

| | LPM | \multicolumn{5}{c}{Time in Hours} |
		1	2	3	4	5
Pressure Gauge Reading	2200 psi	115	57	38	28	23
	200 psi	104	52	34	26	20
	1800 psi	94	47	31	23	18
	1600 psi	83	41	27	20	16
	1400 psi	73	36	24	18	14
	1200 psi	62	33	20	15	12
	1000 psi	52	26	17	13	10
	800 psi	41	21	13	10	8
	600 psi	31	15	10	7	6

Adapted from Using your oxygen cylinder system, Abbey Foster Medical Corporation, 1988, Home Health Care Division.

How to Read the Chart

1. Read pressure gauge on the cylinder
2. Determine liter flow per minute
3. Find the appropriate flow rate on the top
4. Read down the chart to the approximate pressure reading
5. Read the approximate time left in O_2 cylinder at the same liter flow.

NOTE: Do not allow the cylinder pressure to fall below 500 psi because the client may run out of oxygen

Calculating Time for Oxygen Cylinders
E Cylinder

Pressure on cylinder gauge (PSI)
500 psi (safety margin) $\times$ .3 (E cylinder factor) $\div$ LPM = minutes

H Cylinder

Pressure on cylinder gauge (PSI)
500 psi (safety margin) $\times$ 3.1 (H cylinder factor) $\div$ LPM = minutes

Liquid Oxygen

LPM	Stationary Reservoirs		Portable Units	
	17,000 L	25,000 L	500 L	1000 L
1	248 hr	396 hr	7 hr	14 hr
2	124 hr	198 hr	3 hr	7 hr
3	83 hr	134 hr	2 hr	4 hr/30 min
4	61 hr	99 hr	1 hr/30 min	3 hr/30 min
5	40 hr	80 hr	—	—
6			1 hr	2 hr

INDEX